sability

Charles Seale-Hayne Library
University of Plymouth
(01752) 588 588
LibraryandITenquiries@plymouth.ac.uk

For Elsevier:

Commissioning Editor: Dinah Thom
Development Editor: Catherine Jackson
Project Manager: Emma Riley
Designer: George Ajayi
Cartoonist: David Banks

Understanding Disability

A Guide for Health Professionals

Sally French DipGradPhys DipTP BSc(Hons) MSc(Psych) MSc(Soc) PhD
Associate Lecturer, Open University

John Swain BSc(Hons) PGCE MSc PhD
Chair of Disability and Inclusion, School of Health, Welfare and Education, Northumbria University, Newcastle, UK

Foreword by
Frances Reynolds PhD BSc DipPsychCouns
Reader in Psychology, School of Health Sciences and Social Care, Brunel University, London, UK

CHURCHILL
LIVINGSTONE

ELSEVIER

EDINBURGH LONDON NEW YORK OXFORD PHILADELPHIA ST LOUIS SYDNEY TORONTO 2008

CHURCHILL
LIVINGSTONE
ELSEVIER

© 2008, Elsevier Limited. All rights reserved.

First published 2008

ISBN: 978 0 443 10139 7

British Library Cataloguing in Publication Data
A catalogue record for this book is available from the British Library

Library of Congress Cataloging in Publication Data
A catalog record for this book is available from the Library of Congress

Note
Neither the Publisher nor the Authors assume any responsibility for any loss or injury and/or damage to persons or property arising out of or related to any use of the material contained in this book. It is the responsibility of the treating practitioner, relying on independent expertise and knowledge of the patient, to determine the best treatment and method of application for the patient.

The Publisher

Working together to grow
libraries in developing countries

www.elsevier.com | www.bookaid.org | www.sabre.org

ELSEVIER   BOOK AID International   Sabre Foundation

ELSEVIER   your source for books,
journals and multimedia
in the health sciences

www.elsevierhealth.com

The
Publisher's
policy is to use
**paper manufactured
from sustainable forests**

Printed in China

Contents

Foreword

In this accessible, thought-provoking book, Sally French and John Swain encourage qualified and student therapists (and other health professionals) to think deeply about the needs and aspirations of the disabled people with whom they work. They explore the recurring challenges that people experience when living with long-term illness, physical impairment, mental health problems or learning difficulties. Unusually, they report on the experiences both of disabled service providers as well as service users. Their discussion reveals the skills and resources that disabled people bring to health care, as well as highlighting the ways in which difficulties arise from unexamined oppressive social systems and attitudes.

The book traces historical changes in the professions of physiotherapy and occupational therapy, and the wider social and political forces that influenced how disabled people were treated in the twentieth century. Through reading first-person accounts, readers glimpse lives that were blighted by harsh institutional regimes, and by unpleasant medical therapies imposed without consultation. If not kept out of sight, disabled people all too often found themselves being made physically 'acceptable', even when this acceptability required painful operations, or clumsy prosthetic limbs. Whilst offering a critical perspective, the authors do not hector or blame health professionals for current inadequacies of practice. Instead, readers are invited to identify for themselves the current taken-for-granted assumptions that operate in health care and rehabilitation. The authors discuss the pervasive influence of the biomedical model and its premise that disabled people need 'cure' or 'normalization' in order to live satisfactory lives, as well as the power imbalances in the healthcare system which continue to silence or distort the voice of service users.

The authors present the social model of disability with great clarity, helping readers to understand the barriers that disabled people face in participating fully in everyday life, and maintaining meaningful roles and occupations. Through encountering models of critical reflection, guided activities, as well as research that vividly presents the voices of disabled people, readers will find themselves confronting the complexities of current 'buzzwords' such as empowerment, independence and partnership.

The authors seek to make the field of disability studies accessible for health professionals and relevant to practice, through providing various reflective activities. Greater accessibility is clearly needed. This subject, whilst gathering momentum within academia, appears to have had only marginal impact to date on professional education and perspectives. For example, recent research showing that children with cerebral palsy have as good a quality of life as their peers has been met with surprise by parents, as well as by health professionals. Such reactions perhaps reveal how deeply ingrained is the association between impairment and tragedy within our culture.

Readers are likely to find themselves increasingly aware of the many structural barriers to change within health and social care (and within the wider society) that diminish disabled people's choices and quality of life. Yet the book also carries positive messages that individual therapists can create meaningful change, even within a context of limited time and resources. We learn about what is currently positive within health care and rehabilitation, from the viewpoints of disabled people. These accounts show that person-centred practice is highly valued, and that therapists' communication and relationship-building skills are as important to rehabilitation outcomes as their technical expertise. Some of the communication skills are not difficult to acquire, such as *asking* service users what they need to build a satisfying lifestyle rather than telling them what they need. Yet therapists' existing status and assumptions about their roles create barriers to genuine partnership working. The book carefully avoids empty exhortations but offers engaging activities to help the reader develop not only a better intellectual understanding of disability but useful strategies for working in alliance with clients.

Healthcare and rehabilitation professionals are increasingly expected to use evidence to guide practice. Unfortunately, the evidence which is judged to be most valid tends to be positivistic in nature, overly influenced by the biomedical model of disability, and focused solely upon measurable functional outcomes. The authors show that taken-for-granted 'tragedy' perspectives on disability are also incorporated within many current research tools and methods. One of the chapters in this book offers a refreshing alternative perspective by offering evidence derived from participatory research methods in which disabled people themselves initiate and control the research. The findings of such studies provide many insights into disabled people's needs, aspirations and preferences.

The book is also helpful for introducing student and qualified therapists to the range of resources that are (or should be) available for disabled people, including Independent/Integrated Living Centres which have a user-controlled ethos, thereby avoiding the usual barriers of status and power in traditional services.

In brief, this is a book which offers therapists, and other health professionals, the opportunity to learn about the social and political dimensions of disability and health care, to question existing roles and practice, and to work in more appropriate ways *with*, rather than *on*, disabled people.

Frances Reynolds

Chapter 1

What is critical reflection?

We are not beginning this book as might be expected, by examining the meaning of key terms like disability and impairment. Nor are we leaping into the more usual subject matter of disability studies such as prejudice, inaccessibility and disablist language. We begin, instead, by exploring the possibilities for the engagement of professionals with disability studies, the possibilities for developing professional practice, and the processes of change. We hope that it will be clear by the end of this introductory chapter why this is our starting point.

QUESTIONS, QUESTIONS, QUESTIONING QUESTIONS

You need a notebook, journal or workbook to document your thinking and responses as you read and consider the ideas discussed in this book. Those of you familiar with distance learning, for example with the Open University, may feel comfortable with this approach. This can, however, feel at the best unnecessary (bits to skip) and at the worst threatening (with implications that your thinking and practice are not good enough). We could begin with why you bought, borrowed or stole this book (and who you stole it from!). This is our shared starting point: what are you looking for and how do you wish to use this book? And perhaps the most threatening question – why? We shall end this chapter by considering how you might use this book, but to get there we shall begin by engaging you in the questioning approach. You will consider the first of many questions in the following activity.

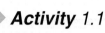

Activity 1.1

WHAT IS GOOD PRACTICE?

Make a few notes to summarize your thoughts on the meaning of 'good practice'.

Did you find this an easy question to answer? As you might expect in a chapter entitled 'What is critical reflection?', we hope that you did not.

The following discussion considers some of the embedded questions inherent in the question, 'What is good practice?' Good practice can be determined and defined within the knowledge base – in recent parlance this is referred to as evidence-based practice. It is good practice because research has shown, for instance, that one form of therapy is better than another. Second, good practice is grounded in the informed intuition, creativity and art of the experienced practitioner. Third, good practice is defined in the evaluation of practice. This can be in the evaluation of process and/or product. In terms of process, notions of good practice can be and are expressed, perhaps derogatively, by 'buzz words', such as partnership, empowerment and client-centred practice. In terms of product, good practice may be defined in terms of meeting the needs, hopes and expectations of clients, and indeed practitioners.

Within these ways of conceiving good practice there are embedded issues relating to how it is defined and who defines it. The question of 'how' relates to science, research and the knowledge base of good practice. If good practice is based on scientific evidence, one line of questioning addresses the quality of the evidence – how valid and reliable is it? This is a much disputed and debated arena. Jupp (2006:250), for instance, suggests quantitative methods of research do not pay attention to social meanings and the ways in which we construct our social world. Qualitative research, based for instance on case studies or the lives and experiences of individuals, provides ground for critical reflection but also raises questions concerning whether the findings can be generalized when considering practice: can good practice be based on the examination of a few cases, particularly when the research cannot be replicated?

As noted above, research-based evidence is not the only knowledge base for practice. Practitioners' knowledge of what constitutes good practice is also founded in practice itself. The idea of reflective practice is grounded in the development of 'practice in action'. This can include ideas of intuition, creativity and problem-solving thinking by practitioners.

Finally, reverberating throughout is the question of *who* defines good practice? This takes us into the realm of political questions and of power relations between the different participants. Such differences in the power to define what is good practice can even be embedded in the terms used to refer to the participants. On one side there are patients, clients, customers, service users, carers and so on, each term connoting a particular relationship between disabled people and service providers. It works in the other direction too of course. Terms such as professional, service provider, care, cure, intervention and even 'practice' have political connotations. Consider the term 'professional', for instance, and its implications for relationships including expertise, the rightful power to define needs, to intervene and to allocate resources. 'Stakeholder' is another current and widely used term that covers all those with an interest in defining good practice – policy makers at national, regional and local levels, academics and researchers, practitioners, service managers, informal carers and disabled people themselves. The term can, however, gloss over real differences in views from different standpoints and obscure possible conflicts. What is 'at stake' depends on the standpoint of stakeholders and there are inequalities between stakeholders in their power to define and determine what is good practice.

In answering the question 'What is good practice?' we have attempted to demonstrate that questions beget questions that it will take us the rest of this book to address. We shall turn first to the development of practice by practitioners, exploring the notion of reflective practice.

REFLECTIVE PRACTICE

There is now a plethora of literature for health professionals that takes a broadly reflective practice approach, though there are differences among the specific models used. There is also an abundance of courses, both pre-service and in-service, that wholly or partly embrace reflective practice. We shall look first at the basic principles of reflective practice and where these ideas come from. We shall then ask for your opinion on the strength of this approach. Finally we will use a research-based example to consider possible limitations. We will begin by looking at a definition of reflective practice. Gould (1996:1) writes:

> There is considerable empirical evidence, based on research into a variety of occupations, suggesting that expertise does not derive from the application of rules or procedures applied deductively from positivist research. Instead, it is argued that practice wisdom rests upon highly developed intuition which can be difficult to articulate but can be demonstrated in practice.

An understanding of professional knowledge as developed by practitioners themselves, through and within their practice and their systematic analysis of practice, is central to the origins of the notion of reflective practice. These ideas have been developed in different ways and in a variety of contexts. Ghaye & Lillyman (2000), for instance, have produced a series of books on reflection for healthcare professionals. They offer a framework of 12 principles of reflection with particular emphasis on the first three (Ghaye & Lillyman 2000:121):

1. Reflective practice is about you and your work.
2. Reflective practice is about learning from experience.
3. Reflective practice is about valuing what we do and why we do it.

The 'father' of these developments is generally acknowledged to be Donald Schön (1983, 1987). In his view (1983:50):

> both ordinary people and professional practitioners often think about what they are doing, sometimes even while doing it … It is this entire process of reflection-in-action which is central to the 'art' by which practitioners deal well with situations of uncertainty, instability, uniqueness and value conflict.

He also stated that (1983:61):

> Practitioners do reflect on their knowledge-in-practice. Sometimes in the relative tranquillity of a post-mortem, they think back on a project they have undertaken, a situation they have lived through, and they explore the understandings they have brought to their handling of the case.

Schön's work has been widely adopted, and adapted, in professional training and development.

So let us get to the crux of this issue and look at a framework for reflective practice presented by Rolfe et al (2001). Their book is a users' guide for nurses and the helping professions. They first distinguish between 'macro' and 'micro' models of reflective practice. Macro models address the underlying philosophy of reflection and possible stages in developing thinking and action. One example of the work they draw on is that of Kim (1999) whose model goes through three phases:

1. Descriptive phase – the practitioner taking a particular situation, event or encounter and asking what happened.
2. Reflective phase – the practitioner asking 'What did I make of this?'
3. Critical/emancipatory phase – the practitioner moving the questioning forward to the implications for acting, thinking and feeling differently.

At the micro level, models address ways in which reflection is conducted and facilitated within each of these phases. This will become clearer in Box 1.1 which summarizes this framework for reflective practice, incorporating both the macro and the micro.

Box 1.1 A framework for reflective practice

Descriptive phase
- What is the problem?
- What was my role in the situation?
- What was I trying to achieve?
- What actions did I take?
- What was the response of others?
- What were the consequences?
- What feelings did it invoke in the client?
- What feelings did it invoke in me?
- What was good/bad about the experience?

Reflective phase
- So what does this tell me?
- So what was going through my mind as I acted?
- So what did I base my actions on?
- So what other knowledge can I bring to the situation?
- So what could I have done to make it better?
- So what is my new understanding of the situation?
- So what broader issues arise from the situation?

Critical/emancipatory phase
- Now what do I need to do in order to stop being stuck?
- Now what broader issues need to be considered if this action is to be successful?
- Now what might be the consequences of this action?

(Derived from Rolfe et al 2001:34–39)

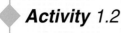

Activity 1.2

REFLECTING ON PRACTICE

The best way to evaluate a reflective approach to the development of practice is to try it out for yourself. Using the questions in the framework for reflective practice (Box 1.1), reflect on a situation you have experienced or a particular problem you have encountered as a practitioner or a student. Reflect on your practice by writing notes in response to each of the questions. Do not worry if some of the questions seem irrelevant to the particular situation you are considering.

Whether or not you were able to carry out the first part of this activity, make a list of what you consider to be the strengths of the reflective practice approach.

(Derived from Ghaye 2000:70–72)

Ghaye (2000) provides a list of the claims of reflective practice that may be useful to compare with your list of strengths. In doing so he uses the plural term 'reflective practices' to emphasize that it covers a number of different approaches rather than just one. There are four claims:

1. Reflective practices improve the quality of care we give.
2. Reflective practices enhance individual and collective professional development.
3. Reflective practices change the power relationship between academics and practitioners by broadening who generates and controls knowledge for safe and competent health care.
4. Reflective practices improve the clinical environment.

Within this claim it is suggested that practitioners need to recognize and be critical of organizational structures that condition and shape professional practice.

Reflective practices also help to build a better world: here it is suggested that reflective practices connect with hopes, intentions and struggles for more just, democratic, compassionate, caring and dignified healthcare systems.

Ghaye & Lillyman also provide a list of the qualities of reflective practice which concentrate more on the personal benefits from the practitioners' viewpoint (2000:36):

- Authenticity: coming to know our authentic self through meaningful relationships with others in our healthcare team and organization.

- Intentionality: where our shared intentions are to act in a systematic, supportive, constructively critical and creative manner in order to enhance practice and the quality of care. This refers to putting our 'heart and soul' into realizing our hopes.

- Sensibility: reflective practitioners are sensitive to their own needs and wants and to the needs and wants of those they work with and care for; reflection heightens our sensitivities.

- Spirituality: reflection can foster a deep sense of obligation, commitment and moral purpose to our work. Through our caring practices, we appreciate a sense of connectedness and mutual interdependence with those for whom we care. Through reflection we experience a sense of being part of, and connected to, something larger and more significant than 'the self'.

Activity 1.3

LIMITATIONS OF REFLECTIVE PRACTICE

We turn now to possible limitations of reflective practice, at least as conveyed above. To do so we shall draw on a small-scale study we undertook which was written into a chapter for a book we edited for therapists working with people with learning difficulties (Swain & French 1999). We approached three groups of people inviting them to participate, and then sent them each a copy of the audiotaped summary of the chapter and a blank audiotape for them to record and return their opinions. The three groups were occupational therapists (OT), physiotherapists (P) and a group of people with learning difficulties (PLD) who worked together as researchers. Below we give a summary of participants' opinions about participation and partnership.

As you read, return again to the framework for reflective practice (Box 1.1) and think about the implications in terms of possible limitations of this approach, though recognizing that reflective practice is not a single approach (Ghaye 2000).

PARTICIPATION

The first topic is participation, and the support and intervention required to enable people with learning difficulties to live and participate as full and active members of the community. The main issues in the discussion of the people with learning difficulties in relation to participation concerned their experiences of, first, segregation:

PLD: I went to BM, boarding school, I couldn't understand why … When I went to boarding school I thought you were being locked up for the rest of your life … I was pushed from one school to other schools, and I ended up in BM.

and, second, barriers that limit participation in inclusive settings, including expectations, lack of support, attitudes and prejudice:

PLD: I go to college and people say to me, 'Why do you want to do level 2?' I say to them, 'I want to get more qualifications.' Because if you do a higher job you get better pay.

PLD: People have been saying to me 'You can't do that', and I say 'Why not?' And they say 'I think you are going to get really tired', and I say 'I'm not'. That is what I want to do, that is what my aim is.

PLD: Anybody with learning disability needs support. You can't just go into a research group, like what we were talking about, without thinking what support do I need, when do I need it?

PLD: Some people just laugh at you and think it is funny.

Occupational therapists also discussed barriers to participation, concentrating on the denial of opportunities particularly in families:

OT: People manage very well really. Saying that though, one thing that I find quite a challenge is when somebody's referred to you and this person's got a lot more abilities than they've ever been allowed to use. That they could be a lot more independent, but they have this role in the family of being 'the child' and the parents do everything for them.

For physiotherapists the problems of integration were predominant:

P: Inclusive schooling for those with a profound disability will need enormous funding in terms of having the right level of assistance in the classroom to enable that person to get the most out of their schooling. Even within policies at the moment of trying to integrate, quite rightly so, physical disability, they struggle. We know teachers who are really struggling with knowing what to do with the more profoundly disabled child because they haven't got enough staffing levels.

PARTNERSHIP

So what did the three groups have to say about partnership? The physiotherapists specifically discussed the notion of partnership in their work with clients with learning difficulties. Though they were generally in favour of negotiation with clients in practice, they also wanted the notion of partnership to include others, and argued that there were limitations to partnerships:

P: I'm hoping that the chapter does highlight that often you're working in partnership with carers and other people involved with the client as well as the clients themselves. It's interesting that they brought up the ethical issue of informed consent; much discussion has gone on here in terms of when you've got a child with a profound disability then it's quite easy to get informed consent from parents, but once they are post-18 there are decisions that you feel the parents aren't making appropriately that you need a multidisciplinary team decision on it. That's an enormous issue, particularly when you've got people who can't speak for themselves.

P: Perhaps it's even more difficult when you've got a client who is capable of communicating but is not fully able to understand what they're dealing with. Perhaps our clients who are profoundly handicapped and can't have a voice for themselves are almost better off because they don't have to make a decision whereas there are clients who fall between two stools, they can perhaps talk to you and hold a conversation but they might not necessarily be able to assimilate knowledge to make an adequate informed choice.

The occupational therapists also saw partnership as 'good practice' and an ideal that they promoted. Like the physiotherapists, they discussed the barriers to partnership but from a different standpoint. For physiotherapists, the main concerns seemed to lie with the limitations of the client in terms of capacities to communicate and understand, whereas the occupational therapists focused on the constraints they faced in realizing the ideal of partnership.

OT: I know we have this philosophy but I do wonder how empowered we are to make some of these things work. It's lip service to a lot of things. You need to involve service managers. I was thinking about abuse. I mean people are abused all the time aren't they, by not giving them choice, not giving them time to do something they enjoy doing, making decisions, taking away their independence and doing things for them. People think that because people are out in the community things are much better but it's not good enough yet, is it? I certainly get quite frustrated as an OT; you suggest something and people just won't take it on board.

OT: I don't know about you but listening to this I think 'Yes, I try to be all these things', but I don't know how much I do because it's really, really difficult to empathize: we can think of what it might be like to have a severe learning disability and to be in a wheelchair, but there is a power struggle; we are the people 'doing' and they are the people being 'done to'. They don't get the chance to do enough.

The group of people with learning difficulties did not use the term 'partnership'. They had a broad discussion about their experiences, emphasizing choices, rights and being listened to.

PLD: Yes, I got my own life to lead.

PLD: It's my choice about who I want to live with.

PLD: But most people don't get what they want really. It depends.

PLD: But people with learning difficulties have their rights.

PLD: Depends who wants to listen to you. This block in this chapter, I think it's a great idea, people listening to you, and why they listen to you, for different reasons. It might be disability reasons, maybe for housing reasons, caring reasons. They're there to listen to you, and care is a big thing in this.

There seem to us to be some significant differences between the standpoints of the three groups. For instance, whereas the people with learning difficulties talked of the difficulties of segregation, physiotherapists talked of the difficulties of integration. The main issue that arises for us is that, given the different standpoints, reflective practice does not necessarily address power relations between service users and service providers. While it may be used to do so, it is not an inherent part of the process. Looking again at the questions in the framework for reflective practice (Box 1.1), from the outset it would seem that it is the professionals' problems that are being addressed. The viewpoint of the client is given some recognition, in the question 'What feelings did it invoke in the client?' but only as defined by, and taken into account by, the professional. You may have noticed that Ghaye's (2000) list of claims of reflective practices cites changing academic–practitioner power relations, but not practitioner–service user power relations. It could even be argued that, rather than challenging service provider–user power relations, reflective practice could justify and strengthen power inequalities inasmuch as clients are subjected to ostensibly well-grounded 'good practice' founded in a reflective approach. Furthermore, 'broader issues' are only referred to in the final question in the framework. The broader issues of discrimination faced by disabled people, and the policy and organizational constraints faced by professionals, are not central and, by implication at least, are put in abeyance.

The unequal power relationship between service providers and service users will be a theme that we shall turn to repeatedly as it is deeply ingrained within the service system. Through reflective practice professionals can aspire to 'connect with hopes, intentions and struggles for more just, democratic, compassionate, caring and dignified healthcare systems' (Ghaye 2000:72).

Overall, reflective practice asks many questions about professional practice, as you can see in Box 1.1. Nevertheless, professionals generate the questions and it can be argued that reflective practice does not inherently question the questions. So let us turn to the broader context and see where this leads us.

A BROADER CONTEXT

Here we shall briefly consider two models or frameworks of critical reflection that attempt to address broader questions of good practice. In doing so we are looking towards still wider questioning, particularly given the possible limitations of reflective practice outlined above.

In the volume edited by Brechin et al (2000), critical reflection is incorporated into a broader idea of critical practice. Brechin (2000:26) explains:

> The term 'critical' is used here to refer to open-minded, reflective appraisal that takes account of different perspectives, experiences and assumptions.

Processes of empowerment and anti-oppression are seen as crucial. She picks out two overall guiding principles. The first is the principle of 'respecting others as equals'. This is justified, in part, by the 'endemic oppression of less powerful groups in society' (2000:31). The second guiding principle is openness. This is an acceptance that there is a degree of uncertainty in all professional practice and that professional practice is evolving within the particular social and historical context. Dewey (1933:29) defined openness as follows:

> Active desire to listen to more sides than one, to give heed to facts from whatever source they come, to give full attention to alternative possibilities, to recognise the possibility of error even in the beliefs that are dearest to us.

Founded on these principles, Brechin (2000) goes on to outline three pillars of critical practice: forging relationships, seeking to empower others and making a difference.

In our previous work (Swain et al 2004a) we also developed a framework of principles, which shares many of the elements of Brechin's model and attempts to incorporate critical reflection within a broader context of enabling relationships, empowerment and emancipation. It is summarized in Box 1.2.

Box 1.2 An enabling relationships framework of principles

Critical reflection
1. To promote understanding of self and others through personal reflection and through dialogue.
2. To facilitate functional reflection through critical examination of the practice/process of therapy to reveal its assumptions, values and biases.
3. To develop disciplinary reflection and a critical stance towards therapy within broader debates about theory and practice.

Enabling relationships
4. To promote mutual understanding and awareness of others' preferences, wishes and needs through open two-way communication.

5. To facilitate, through working in partnership, a collaborative approach to service organization, planning, delivery and evaluation.

Empowerment and emancipation

6. To facilitate the recognition and questioning of power relations, structures and ideologies that limit people's freedom.
7. To promote people's prediction and control over decision-making processes that shape their lives.
8. To promote people's struggles against oppression and 'man-made' sufferings, support the removal of barriers to equal opportunities and promote full participatory citizenship for all.

(Derived from Swain et al 2004a:90–91, with permission from Elsevier)

Activity 1.4

A SERVICE USER'S EXPERIENCE

At this point let us look in some detail at the experiences of a disabled person as a service user: Arlene. Occupational therapy in housing was the specific focus of the interview and it comes from a small-scale piece of research (French & Swain 2006). As you read about Arlene's experiences, return again to the question 'What is good practice?' Use the enabling relationships framework of principles shown in Box 1.2. Tick off, or make notes about, the principles that are directly, or indirectly, important to Arlene's experiences.

My first experience with occupational therapists ... was after I was given the wheelchair in hospital when I was in for that year. I was in the middle of doing my OU degree and studied from my bed because I was in my bed more often when I was in hospital. I got pushed, because I didn't have my powerchair, to the occupational therapy department one day and they said to me, did I want to make a cake or make a basket. I didn't want to do either and I said 'What else?' and she said, 'No you can either make a cake or make a basket or you can fry an egg' – that was the other thing they suggested. And I thought, I have no interest in doing this and I would rather be doing what I was doing in the first place, which was reading my book. They didn't think I had any need to do any sort of study. As a disabled person I wasn't going to be able to cope with cooking and things within my home environment ... They were treating me like a child as well and I didn't like the feeling. And then they decided that they would come and assess my new home environment, but they didn't take me, so it wasn't until well into the adaptations that the occupational therapists said, 'Oh we ought to go visit with you.' And at that point the accessible kitchen, I realized, was inaccessible ... because they hadn't measured it in my power wheelchair, which I was going to have; they had measured a standard manual chair.

They had also decided to put in a gas hob and gas oven, and oxygen-dependent people shouldn't be near a naked flame, so for three years, because of the occupational therapists' neglect ... I was unable to use the kitchen at all. They also hadn't considered the fact that when I came out of hospital I was going to be in bed a lot of the time because I've got brittle bones as well and my legs at that point were damaged and I couldn't get to answer the door and I had to fight to get an intercom system put in so I could open the door. So for about the first three years that I lived here, despite arguing with the occupational therapists that it was dangerous, my front door stood open and they said 'You can have a dog because the dog will bark if someone comes in.' Which is wonderful because I like animals but the dog was so small at that time. It was a Yorkshire terrier. I couldn't imagine my Yorkshire terrier being able to frighten anybody off. And it was only after I had somebody come into the flat who, it was like a conman type thing and he was in the flat and he was appraising what he could swipe, that they decided that I could have an intercom and open the door.

A lot of occupational therapists haven't got any knowledge of what it's like to be disabled ... they've done a course at university therefore they think that they know it all ... I've only met one OT that's any good ... At first she was a bit wary of me and I was definitely wary of her ... we got on really well because she actually listened to me and that made the difference.

First, we suspect you found Arlene's stories challenging, particularly for occupational therapists. She does not pull her punches and is very dissatisfied with the services she has received. Before addressing the question set for the above activity, let's recognize some of the questions or objections that can be raised about the evidence base that these stories present, and have been raised by professionals in our experience:

- Are Arlene's experiences typical? Are they generalizable in terms of the experiences of disabled service users? This is a 'typical' objection to qualitative evidence. These might be the particular, even unique, experiences of one service user within a specific 'one-off' context.

- Another objection might be that this is just Arlene's version of events. What were the professionals' experiences and views about what was happening? One strand of this objection is the lack of recognition of professionals' good intentions. From this line of thinking, the word 'allegedly' could be used to qualify Arlene's criticisms of the services she has received.

- A third possible question is whether the criticisms are generalizable to the work of other health and social care professionals. Do Arlene's stories relate solely to the work of occupational therapists or do the implications reverberate across service user–provider relations?

- A final objection that might be posed is that professional practice has developed. There is no recognition in Arlene's stories that professional policy, practice and provision is changing.

While such objections can fuel discussion, and it is legitimate to question the basis of the evidence being considered, they are problematic. Basically they are a way of dismissing Arlene's views and experiences, as the professionals who worked with her, indeed, generally dismissed them. The fundamental challenge at the heart of the stories is being avoided. The challenge is that the apparent solutions provided by professional services can themselves become the problems. Good intentions can pave the road to hell. The more positive response is to consider the implications for good practice.

Looking back at the enabling relationships framework of principles, many if not all the principles are at least implied in Arlene's stories. Some points are, however, repeatedly highlighted. We would pinpoint the following:

- Arlene's stories are centrally about the broader context of the power relations between service users and providers. The development of good practice is centrally dependent on changing these power relations. This reinforces the points made in the previous activity.

- The emphasis throughout is on service providers listening to disabled people. Her stories are about not being consulted and listened to, and the consequences of not being listened to. They are also about her struggles to have her needs, as she sees them, taken into account. If there is a key message for professionals in developing good practice, it is the need to listen.

- Associated with this are her struggles against professionals' presumptions about herself, her life and her needs. These are the presumptions of 'the expert' who assesses problems and provides solutions – and defines good practice within the process. Within Arlene's stories the solutions become the problems and good practice involves challenging expert presumptions.

- It is also apparent that good practice is determined within the practice of individual practitioners and the service system: the efficiency of practice. Specifically, within Arlene's stories, this would include the provision of equipment that does what it is supposed to do and within a reasonable timescale.

- Finally, there are implications for interpersonal relationships between service users and providers. The delivery of good practice is embedded in the quality of relationships.

So far we have focused on Arlene's experiences of service provision under the umbrella topic of housing in terms of accessibility and independent living within her home. We selected the above extracts from her interview that directly addressed this topic. Looking at the broader context, however, in Arlene's stories questions of housing went well beyond the comfort and practicalities of living within her home. First there is the immediate context. Arlene has been subject to abuse by her neighbours living in the building where she has her flat. She was, for instance, forced into using the back door to the building rather than the front. Second, think of all the factors that you took into account when choosing where to live – local shops, local amenities, distance to travel to work and so on. Housing cannot be examined in isolation as it is linked to access to all the community facilities (Esmond et al 1998). After becoming impaired Arlene had no choice over where she lived. Furthermore, there are major problems for Arlene in accessing the local environment to the extent that she is, in this respect, confined to her home. She overcomes this by having her own transport, an adapted van, which she uses to travel to more accessible amenities. Third, housing issues for Arlene need to be seen in the general context of lack of accessible housing for disabled people. As Imrie (1998:129) states:

> Western cities are characterised by a design apartheid where building form and design are inscribed into the values of an 'able-bodied' society … This has led some commentators to regard the built environment as disablist, that is projecting 'able-bodied' values which legitimate oppressive and discriminatory practices against disabled people purely on the basis that they have physical and mental impairments.

Arlene cannot, for instance, access the house where her mother lives. She visits her mother but her mother has to come to Arlene's van to see her. She told us how this affects her social life generally. Friends have to visit her rather than her visiting friends. Furthermore, there is little or no possibility for Arlene of finding another home adapted to her requirements. Broadening the context, then, Arlene's stories are of the disabling society, the discrimination faced by people with impairments who do not conform to the norms of the non-disabled society.

To engage in critical reflection is to engage with the disabling society in which we all live and to engage with people's lives within the disabling society. It is this that we shall be exploring within this book, and we shall turn next to how we hope to do this.

HOW TO USE THIS BOOK

It is usual for the first chapter of a book of this type to provide you, the reader, with guidelines on how to approach or use the book, given that it is written with a workbook approach. We have already attempted to engage you in the process before making specific suggestions in the hope that it will be more meaningful at this point. The aim of the book is to:

engage you in critically reflecting on professional policy, provision and practice from a disability studies standpoint.

Disability studies is the basis that we shall be developing for critical reflection in this book. As we hope has become apparent throughout this introductory chapter, this is not a simple process. Disability studies will not provide a 'cookbook' of predetermined recipes for good practice. As approached in this book it is first and foremost a questioning process, and questions beget questions. What are the most helpful questions? Who determines the questions? How are questions determined? As you may have noted, the title of most of the chapters in this book are in the form of questions.

This book has, therefore, been designed as a book to be worked through as well as simply read. At various points within each chapter you will find activities that are aimed at helping you get the most out of the ideas being discussed. There are a number of processes that can be effective and can be drawn on in facilitating critical reflection. We shall outline two: reflective writing and collaboration.

This notion of reflective writing is summarized by Rolfe et al (2001:70) as follows:

> … the reflective writing process is a way of making connections between previously disparate pieces of information, of developing ways of organising or reorganising thoughts, and of exploring issues and structures so as to be able to take a new perspective on them.

Writing, in this sense, is an active engagement with ideas, a questioning of ideas, a sorting and resorting, thinking and rethinking. The activities are prompts, not tests! How you respond is essentially up to you, though wherever relevant we shall provide our responses.

The second strategy is collaboration; working with others through the book. This might be a single partner, possibly a colleague, with whom you can engage in the activities, or a series of partners with whom to engage as relevant throughout the book. For us, writing is a collaborative, relational activity, and we are suggesting that reading might be the same for you. The more knowledge and experience is pooled, the richer will be the process of learning about human relations. Such collaboration incorporates both one-to-one and group situations.

Collaboration requires the establishment of trust in which people can communicate openly and freely. This involves discussion and negotiation around some complex issues relating to ethics and the processes of communication. For instance, there are questions of anonymity and confidentiality to be dealt with in an agreed code of ethics, which might remain informal but be continually reviewed. Other issues include the invasion of privacy, the right to opt out and the establishment of equity in participation so that the group or one-to-one situation is not dominated or manipulated from one side.

Understanding Disability: a Guide for Health Professionals is for physiotherapists and occupational therapists as well as students of these professions. Given the focus on disability studies, however, we hope it will be of relevance and of use for all healthcare workers. This book is also intended for professional and non-professional educators and trainers in the therapy field, and we shall turn to this particular use of the book in the concluding chapter. Overall this book is about the questioning of notions of good practice, developing understanding and challenging taken-for-granted assumptions. It is about possibilities for changing professional policy, provision and practice. It is about an active, reactive, proactive process that links with hopes and struggles for a less disablist and more inclusive society for all.

Chapter 2

What is disability?

In this chapter we will be discussing the meaning of disability by considering various models. This is important because models of disability, or what we think disability is, underlie both policy and practice. The first activities in this chapter are aimed to help you enter these complex debates.

WHAT IS DISABILITY?

Activity 2.1

WHAT DOES DISABILITY MEAN TO YOU?

Write down a few words and phrases that, for you, convey the meaning of the word 'disability'.

   The purpose of this question is for you to verbalize your thinking about disability. It provides a basis for your personal reflections as you progress through the book. We will be asking you the same question later on. At this stage your answer will depend on many factors, for instance whether or not you consider yourself to be disabled and your experiences with disabled people.

◆ *Activity* 2.2

WHO IS DISABLED?

One of us (John) has diabetes. Is John disabled? Why do you consider him to be disabled – or not disabled?

Is a person with a facial disfigurement disabled? In thinking about this, read the following extracts from Vicky Lucas's story. Is Vicky disabled? Why do you consider Vicky disabled – or not disabled?

I have a rare genetic disorder called Cherubism, which affects my face. I was diagnosed when I was about four years old. I was too young to remember what happened, but visiting hospitals became a regular part of my life.

Although it was only when I was about six that my face started to really change shape, I don't remember a time when I didn't look different …

My teenage years were difficult. People would sometimes stare or do a double take. Some people would be downright nasty and call me names.

Even when people said 'Oh you poor thing!' their pity also hurt me and that hurt would stay with me for a long time. I became very withdrawn, afraid of how I might be treated if I went out.

But over time I gradually started to develop my self-esteem and self-confidence and I started to feel that I shouldn't waste my life just because of other people's attitudes towards me.

At the age of sixteen I went to college and studied subjects such as film, media studies and photography. I started to research the representation of disfigured people in the media.

When I looked at how people with facial disfigurements are portrayed in films, well, no wonder people don't know how to react to us! Freddy Krueger in *Nightmare on Elm Street*, the Joker in *Batman*, the various scarred villains in gangster films … the list is endless.

With stereotypes like that, it's hardly surprising that people assume that if you have a facial difference, there must be something 'different' or 'bad' about you on the inside too.

This was a huge turning point for me because I realised that facial disfigurement was not just a medical issue, but a social issue as well.

I realised that the reason why I was so unhappy was not because of my face, but the way some people would react to it. I decided that it wasn't my face I wanted to change, but social attitudes …

… my face is integral to who I am. The way people treat me and the way I've had to learn to live my life has created the person I am today.

(Lucas 2003:4–5)

We shall summarize some of our thinking behind these questions.

There are a number of criteria you might have used in considering whether John is disabled:

1. The first is severity of impairment. This way of thinking is based on the idea that whether a person is disabled depends on the degree of the person's impairment. For instance, John is also shortsighted.

Is that sufficient grounds to be deemed disabled? Shortsighted people are not usually considered to be disabled, partly because the impairment is overcome by the use of glasses. So does the same apply to diabetes, and the use of insulin to control sugar levels? It could be argued that if John's diabetes is well controlled he is not disabled, but if it is not well controlled then he is.

2. Official definitions are another criterion. Thus John is disabled if, for instance, diabetes is considered a disability in the Disability Discrimination Act (1995). Similarly a person with a visual impairment, who is registered blind or partially sighted, may be considered disabled, but a person with a visual impairment who is not registered may be considered non-disabled. It is interesting that, by this criterion, who is considered disabled alters with changes in legislation. For instance, until the 1944 Education Act there was no such thing (officially) as partial sight. Also, before that Act the definition of 'blind' was different in employment legislation and education legislation, so it was possible to be blind and then not to be blind (French et al 2006).

3. A third criterion is personal identification. If John identifies himself as being disabled does that mean he is? If not, is he non-disabled? Most people with impairments do not identify themselves as being disabled. Are they therefore non-disabled?

4. A fourth criterion is the social consequences of impairment. Is John disabled if there are social consequences to having diabetes? This takes us into the next question.

People with facial disfigurements are primarily disabled through the responses of others. The main criterion here is social difference in relation to cultural norms and values – in this case socially constructed ideals of beauty. Social difference can, indeed, be seen as playing a role in defining disability, but how far would you go? For instance, do you think a woman who is overweight is disabled? There is certainly similar reasoning. Fat women can face social rejection and be stared at, and there are also stereotypes ingrained in media images. This begs the question of whether social difference is a sufficient criterion for defining disability. For instance, are men with short stature or left-handed people disabled?

A related question is whether people with impairments are disabled in all circumstances. A man with a visual impairment who had formed relationships over citizen-band radio and the Internet, where he deliberately did not identify himself as a disabled person, brought this to the fore for us. This is sometimes referred to as 'passing' for non-disabled, perhaps particularly for people with 'hidden' impairments. Some people with epilepsy, for instance, can, for understandable reasons such as when they apply for employment, pass as non-disabled. This, of course, does not apply only to disabled people. Older women can pass as younger than they are and young people as older, gay and lesbian people can pass as heterosexual, all for understandable reasons. The possibility of passing also gives rise to the possible affirmation of identity by 'coming out'. Inherent within the question of 'What is disability?', then, are questions of identity.

We have used these activities to help raise complex and far-reaching questions that arise in defining disability and the associated question of who is disabled. As you may have noted, even in setting such questions there are underlying presumptions. There may be an inherent pre-sumption that there are two categories of people: disabled and non-disabled. There may be an inherent presumption, too, that disability defines a person's identity. No one, however, is *just* disabled. People are also young or old, male or female, white or members of ethnic minority communities, heterosexual or gay or lesbian, all of which suggest that divisions between people are flexible, fluid and changing, rather than fixed binary categories (Vernon & Swain 2002).

It can also be argued that the question of who is disabled is itself a politically based question. It detracts us from the issues that matter to disabled people, such as what and who create a disabling environment and how environmental barriers can be dismantled? It is clear that we need to stand back from the question of who is disabled to consider other questions, for instance who decides who is disabled, against what criteria such decisions are made, and why?

There are many purposes behind definitions of disability, including the following:

- To count heads – to discover, for instance, how many disabled people there are in the UK.
- To allot resources – to discover what services are needed and who should be entitled to receive them.
- To develop the expertise and knowledge of experts, for instance professionals and policy makers.
- To research disability issues.
- To develop policy in relation to disability.
- To challenge the discrimination, prejudice and oppression faced by disabled people.
- To develop or affirm the collective and individual identity of dis-abled people.

Overall, then, the question 'What is disability?' is a political one. There are deeply ingrained vested interests here. In current parlance, there are stakeholders, and what is 'at stake' is far broader than a simple definition of disability: professionals' jobs, professional status, values and beliefs, social power and control, social identity and disabled people's day-to-day lives are all implicated. You might like to look back at the above list of possible purposes of defining disability and consider which are primarily expressions of the vested interests of service providers, which are primarily the vested interests of disabled people, and where there may be shared interests. These issues are all addressed throughout the following chapters. In this chapter we enter the debates and controversies by exploring the key competing understandings and standpoints towards disability.

WHAT IS THE PROBLEM?

Activity 2.3

WHERE DOES THE PROBLEM LIE?

Look at the following cartoon and make a few notes on what you think is 'the problem' being depicted.

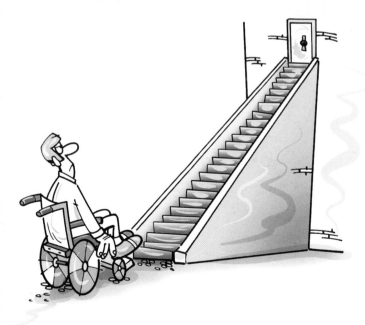

(From Porter 2005 Dictionary of Physiotherapy, Oxford, Elsevier, 95)

The purpose of this activity is to introduce you to two main ways of thinking about disability. This is captured within the following quotation by Finkelstein (1972:8). He is not talking about the cartoon directly, but rather about his own experience of the situation depicted within the cartoon.

Now, an alternative way of looking at this is to say that the cause of disability has got nothing to do with the physical defect of the person at all but it is related to the way that society is organised in relation to that particular physical condition. For example: I can't use my legs, and when I come to a building which has some steps then I can't climb the steps – I can't go into the building because I am disabled. This is the usual way that such a situation might be interpreted; but this is not at all how I might interpret the situation: as the disabled person, the person with the problem, might look at it. The way that I see it is that there are some steps which 'prevent' me from entering the building: it is the steps that cause my disability! It is the barrier in the environment that is making things go wrong.

There are, then, two interpretations of this cartoon and of disability. Either the problem lies within the person so is viewed through an individual model, or the problem lies within the environment so is understood within a social model of disability. Looking at your notes for this activity, words or phrases that trace the problem to the person express an individual model, such as inability to walk or being 'wheelchair-bound' (the latter being a common but erroneous notion as people are not 'bound' to their wheelchairs). A focus on the environment, such as the design of the building or steps as barriers, is an expression of a social model way of thinking.

THE INDIVIDUAL MODEL OF DISABILITY

This book, and indeed the field of disability studies, is underpinned by the social model of disability, though this does not assume unquestioning acceptance of this way of thinking. Disability studies is an arena of controversial issues and debates – and this, for us, is crucial to its strength and vibrancy. Before looking at the social model of disability, let us consider the individual model. Some argue, though not all as we shall see below, that the social and individual model are direct opposites. There is not one easily defined individual model. It is a way of thinking that reverberates through the dominant ways of conceptualizing disability within our society.

Activity 2.4

WHAT IS A MEDICAL MODEL OF DISABILITY?

The main professional version of the individual model is widely referred to as the medical model. Read the following quotations and list what you regard as the key characteristics or assumptions of the medical model.

According to the classic medical notion of disability, disability is the result of a physical condition, is intrinsic to the individual (it is part of that individual's own body), may reduce the individual's quality of life and causes clear disadvantages. Furthermore, a compassionate or just society will put resources into trying to cure disabilities medically or to improve functioning, and the medical profession has a major responsibility and potential for helping disabled people. The medical model of disability is often cited by disabled people's civil rights groups when evaluating the costs and benefits of invasive or traumatic medical procedures, prosthetics, 'cures', and medical tests such as genetic screening or pre-implantation genetic diagnosis. Often, a medical model of disability is used to justify large investment in these procedures, technologies and research ... (www.answers.com)

Indeed, a way of thinking that has come to be called the 'medical model' offers a clarity about how problems at one level can cause difficulties at other levels. Medical practices, organized around the medical model, presume that the physician's task is to diagnose diseases, to discover their causes and symptoms, and design treatments. The treatments are aimed at eliminating or minimizing the symptoms of the disease, or the cause of the disease, or the disease itself. The medical model is made up of causal chains, of primary, secondary, and tertiary causes. The primary cause is often seen as the original cause. It is often depicted as a problem at the biological level. Germs cause the flu, brain damage from accidents or strokes causes communication disabilities. The symptoms of diseases are often cast in psychological terms. Brain damage can cause problems in understanding and producing language. A final link in the causal chain is usually seen as a social one – a language problem causes a person to withdraw from social situations or be excluded from them by others. (Duchan 2001)

We would recognize, first, that these could not be taken as definitive statements. Nevertheless, the features that emerge can be said to characterize the model. We would pick out the following:

- It is predominantly from the standpoint of professionals.
- It underpins and rationalizes professionals' status as experts.
- It underlies the medical industry and the scientific search for cures and treatments.
- It is rationalized as providing the basis for a humane societal response to disability.

- It defines disability as being located within the individual, as a problem, abnormality and the source of unacceptable suffering.
- Impairment is seen as underlying the disabled person's lifestyle and quality of life, such as social isolation and dependency.

A second individual model, which is closely related to the medical model, is the tragedy model. Throughout history and in most cultures disabled people have been viewed as inferior, dangerous, tragic, pathetic and not quite human. This view is dominant, prevalent and infused throughout media representations, language, cultural beliefs, research, policy and professional practice. In relation to language, for instance, 'suffering/sufferer' is perhaps the most widely used terminology in tragedy discourses to characterize the experience of disability.

Activity 2.5

TRAGIC CHARACTERS?

Many non-disabled people will have had little experience on a day-to-day basis of being with disabled people. The images they form about disabled people can be largely based on experiences such as those portrayed through the mass media, particularly television and film. Barnes (1992) has written on this subject and places the portrayals of disabled people in the mass media into ten categories, which construct the notion of tragedy in different ways. As you read, note down examples of characters from the media, films, television programmes or literature which might be thought to portray each of these stereotypes of disabled people.

1. As pitiable and pathetic.
2. As an object of violence.
3. As sinister and evil.
4. As atmosphere or curio.
5. As super cripple.
6. As an object of ridicule.
7. As their own worst and only enemy.
8. As a burden.
9. As sexually abnormal.
10. As incapable of participating fully in community life.

There are numerous examples portraying each of these images of disability. The following are our suggestions:

1. *As pitiable and pathetic: A Christmas Carol* (a book by Charles Dickens which was also made into a film) included two disabled characters.

The best known is the pitiable and pathetic Tiny Tim whose tragedy of using a crutch is miraculously overcome at the end of the film when he runs to meet the enlightened Scrooge. The other is a blind man, with both a dog and a white stick, who appears as a beggar. In the final scene, the humanized Scrooge donates money in the proffered hat, for which the tragic figure of the cap-in-hand (handicapped) blind man is clearly grateful.

2. *As an object of violence:* A woman knows the identity of a murderer. The murderer knows and is stalking her. How might the woman's situation be made more threatening and perilous? One way, as in the film *Spiral Staircase*, is for her to be blind.

3. *As sinister and evil: It's a Wonderful Life* is a film which is widely celebrated for the general sentiments it portrays. It features just one disabled character, Mr Potter, who is rich, evil, twisted, frustrated and in a wheelchair. No other explanation for his inhumanity, which includes theft, is offered other than his response to a life as a wheelchair user (despite the fact that he is, ironically, the richest man in the town). It is the tragedy that has twisted him. The only other evil character, a minor character, in the film is the man who pushes the wheelchair. The tragedy, it seems, begets evil even by association.

4. *As atmosphere or curio:* A newly married couple are on honeymoon in Transylvania. It is night time and foggy, and the car breaks down. They approach a huge sinister house and knock at the door. Who opens the door to Dracula's house? Of course, it is a 'dwarf' or 'hunchback' (to use the associated language).

5. *As super cripple:* 'Supercrips' (named as such by disabled people) are characters that overcome their impairments in what are perceived to be amazing and brave ways. It is sometimes called the 'Douglas Bader syndrome', after the character (based on a real person) who lost his legs in the film *Reach for the Sky*.

6. *As an object of ridicule:* Disabled people are often portrayed as ridiculous, laughable characters. They fall over, fail to understand and generally cause havoc. The cartoon character Mr Magoo, who is visually impaired, is an example.

7. *As their own worst and only enemy:* Lois Keith, in her study of disabled children in literature, talks of characters in post-1970 novels as follows (2001:206):

> Particularly in the weaker stories of this period, the 'handicapped children' in novels often suffered from internalised oppression,

hating themselves, believing that the problems they faced were all their fault and dreaming of how happy they would be if only they could walk.

As their own worst enemies, they do not fit with expectations of cheerfully accepting their lot.

8. *As a burden:* Keith (2001:213) also includes a quotation from a novel by Cordelia Jones (1978) which clearly captures the disabled character as a burden:

Someone who marries a cripple must have something wrong with them. He must need to be indispensable to someone … there's something morbid, unhealthy about wanting to devote the whole of your life to a woman who's crippled. It's not a natural form of love.

9. *As sexually abnormal:* Why did Lady Chatterley (in the novel by D.H. Lawrence, also made into a film and television series) have rampant sex with the gardener? Her husband is a wheelchair user and, it is assumed, cannot gratify her desires and needs.

10. *As incapable of participating fully in community life:* It is always interesting to see what happens to the disabled character by the end of the film, play, television programme or book as he or she almost invariably dies, is cured or is placed within an institution rather than living happily as a disabled person. The film *Rainman* is a good example. Despite having formed a relationship with his brother and demonstrated outstanding abilities, in the last scene he is sent back to the segregated institution he came from.

There are numerous examples you might have selected, including villains in James Bond films and the grocer with a stammer in *Open All Hours.* You might also have noted the lack of presence of disabled actors in films and television programmes as well as disabled presenters and newsreaders.

THE SOCIAL MODEL OF DISABILITY

From the viewpoint of a social model of disability, disability is not caused by a person's impairment; it is the treatment the person receives within a disablist society that causes disability. It is the society that disables people with impairments.

Activity 2.6

WHAT IS A SOCIAL MODEL OF DISABILITY?

Oliver is widely recognized as the first writer to use the term 'social model of disability' though he did so building on considerable developments in thinking already engaged in by disabled people (see Hunt 1966). The following is a more recent statement and, as he has now retired from academic life, one of his final statements on disability. As you read, make a few notes about the social model, as you did in relation to the individual model above.

In the broadest sense, the social model is about nothing more complicated than a clear focus on economic, environmental and cultural barriers encountered by people who are viewed by others as having some form of impairment – whether physical, sensory or intellectual. The barriers disabled people encounter include inaccessible education systems, working environments, inadequate disability benefits, discriminatory health and social support services, inaccessible transport, houses and public buildings and amenities, and the devaluing of disabled people through negative images in the media – films, television and newspapers. Hence, the cultural environment in which we all grow up usually sees impairment as unattractive and unwanted.

(Oliver 2004:21)

The following points are adapted from a statement by the British Council of Disabled People (now called the United Kingdom's Disabled People's Council) (2003):

- The social model was developed by disabled people to help them describe and take action against discrimination.

- The model does not blame the disabled person for the problems he or she has and helps contest internalized oppression.

- Disabled people, by using the social model, can find areas in the world that need changing and find out about bad attitudes towards disabled people, why some people will not talk to disabled people and why disabled people cannot get into some buildings.

- The social model allows disabled people to get together to campaign for better things, like people being considerate towards disabled people, and more access to buildings no matter what the disabled person's impairment is.

- The social model helps disabled people to talk about themselves and about human rights and equality.

- The social model furthers the formation of a collective identity for disabled people.

At this point we look briefly at the sources of the social model. Where did it come from? This is important, as ideas can become disassociated from their roots and in doing so lose their original force.

◆ *Activity 2.7*

WHY A SOCIAL MODEL?

The social model of disability emerged from the disabled people's movement. The following quotations come from research by Campbell & Oliver (1996:30–40) who examined and documented the growth of the movement. What do you think they tell us about the generation of the social model?

It was a specialist hospital and kids and young people came there from all over the country. I was there for nine months with the odd bit of weekend leave and went through an incredible regime of awfulness and torture which they choose to call physiotherapy and such like.

(p. 31)

Well in the earlier days I used to live with my parents. I wasn't allowed to do much even though I was over 18. I wasn't allowed to go out on my own, wasn't allowed to come back on my own, although I was allowed to go out with them if there were celebrations going on but that was a bit boring.

(p. 35)

At that time I did not know any better but they [the doctors] would want to do experimental operations and I let them. I just believed them. I didn't know to resist. I didn't know to say no.

(p. 38)

I've been through special school education. I've been through special college education and at the end of it all I've been rejected ... So I was burning with an anger that I still burn with, but I didn't know how to express it and didn't know where to express it.

(p. 39)

The social model is a tool to challenge, confront and change the disablist society. It arises from disabled people's collective experiences of segregation and institutionalization; enforced isolation and dependency; the domination of the medical model; and the personal and collective 'slow burning anger' that is positively expressed through the social model. Walmsley (2006b:47) points out its considerable success in recent years:

> One could argue that the social model of disability is one of the most significant influences on the philosophical landscape across the whole of social policy in the late twentieth century.

AN AFFIRMATIVE MODEL

It is our contention that an affirmative model is developing out of the individual and collective experiences of disabled people that directly confronts the personal tragedy model, not only of disability but also of impairment. The notion of affirmation is one of great depth – taking us into what we are as human beings. From the documented viewpoint of disabled people, far from being tragic, being disabled can have benefits. There are numerous ways in which disabled people are affirmative that we can only touch upon here.

Activity 2.8

I AM AS I AM?

As you read the following quotations summarize the ways in which you think people are being affirmative of themselves and their lifestyles.

I don't wake up and look at my wheelchair and think 'shit, I've got to spend another day in that', I just get up and get on with it.
(Watson 2002:519)

I will always believe that blindness is a neutral trait, neither to be prized nor shunned.
(Kent 2000:62)

I just can't imagine becoming hearing, I'd need a psychiatrist, I'd need a speech therapist, I'd need some new friends, I'd lose all my old friends, I'd lose my job. I wouldn't be here lecturing. It really hits hearing people that a deaf person doesn't want to become hearing. I am what I am!
(Phillipe in Shakespeare et al 1996:184)

Coming Out

And with the passing of time
you realise you need to find
people with whom you can share.

There's no need to despair.
Your life can be your own
and there's no reason to condone
what passes for their care.
So, I'm coming out.
I've had enough
of passing and playing their game.
I'll hold my head up high.
I'm done with sighs
and shame.

    (Tyneside Disability Arts 1998:35, with permission from Georgina Sinclair)

I do not wish for a cure for Asperger's Syndrome. What I wish for is a cure for the common ill that pervades too many lives, the ill that makes people compare themselves to a normal that is measured in terms of perfect and absolute standards, most of which are impossible for anyone to reach.

    (Holliday Wiley 1999:96)

I am never going to be able to conform to society's requirements and I am thrilled because I am blissfully released from all that crap. That's the liberation of disfigurement.

    (Shakespeare et al 1996:81)

We are not usually snapped up in the flower of youth for our domestic and child rearing skills, or for our decorative value, so we do not have to spend years disentangling ourselves from wearisome relationships as is the case with many non-disabled women.

    (Vasey 1992:74)

As a result of becoming paralysed life has changed completely. Before my accident it seemed as if I was set to spend the rest of my life as a religious sister, but I was not solemnly professed so was not accepted back into the order. Instead I am now very happily married with a home of my own.

    (Morris 1989:120)

Life is very good ... being born with no arms has opened up so many different things that I would never have done. My motto is, 'In life try everything'. I wouldn't have that philosophy if I'd been born with arms.

    (BBC Radio 4 2002)

We are who we are as people with impairments, and might actually feel comfortable with our lives if it wasn't for all those interfering busybodies who feel that it is their responsibility to feel sorry for us, or to find cures for us, or to manage our lives for us, or to harry us in order to make us something we are not, i.e. 'normal'.

    (Tyneside Disability Arts 1999:35)

Sub Rosa

Fighting to establish self-respect ...
Not the same, but different ...

Not normal, but disabled ...
Who wants to be normal anyway?
Not ashamed, with heads hanging,
Avoiding the constant gaze of those who assume
that sameness is something to be desired ...
Nor victims
of other people's lack of imagination ...
But proud and privileged to be who we are ...
Exactly as we are.
>   (Tyneside Disability Arts 1998, with permission from Colin Cameron)

Kondo (1990:48) writes, 'human beings create, construct, work on and enact their identities, sometimes creatively challenging the limits of the cultural constraints.' Affirmation of identity, for us all, is a complex process and can be seen as embedded and inherent within our daily lives and interactions with others. You have only to think, for instance, about the ways in which you affirm, negotiate and also resist a male or female identity to realize some of the intricacies and subtleties of casting and recasting who you are. This is, to an extent, apparent in the above quotations that we interpret as follows:

- Identity is simply a 'fact of life', neither positive nor negative. Given the predominant negative presumptions, such neutrality can itself be a form of resistance or resilience.

- There are clearly positive declarations or affirmations of identity. There is an overturning of the tragedy model here. For most hearing people the notion of becoming deaf is tragic – a perceived loss of capacity to work, to socialize, to listen to music and so on. For Phillipe the tragedy would be to become hearing.

- Life chances as a disabled person are affirmed as against life chances as a non-disabled person. Again the tragedy model is turned on its head, but more in terms of associated lifestyle than personal identity per se. Despite, or in the face of, discrimination and prejudice, life can be full and satisfying.

- Affirmation of identity can be collective as well as individual. There are, of course, parallels with other groups in society. Less clearly political, but nevertheless an example of collective positive affirmation, would be a 'girls' night out'.

WHAT IS DISABILITY IN THERAPY?

This question will be developed and addressed throughout the remaining chapters. At this point an appropriate focus is the knowledge and skills that are developed through therapy training. To engage with training issues we shall look now at disability equality training.

A major strategy to changing disabling behaviours and practices is through the development of disability equality training (DET). Disability equality training was originally devised by disabled people themselves and pioneered by a small group of disabled women in London (particularly by Jane Campbell, Micheline Mason and Kath Gillespie-Sells). In its strict sense, DET originally referred to courses delivered by tutors who had been trained by organizations *of* disabled people, that is organizations run and controlled by disabled people themselves, such as the Disability Resource Team and the Greater Manchester Coalition of Disabled People (Swain et al 1998). These organizations trained disabled people to be trainers. Disability equality training courses are not about changing emotional responses to disabled people but about challenging people's whole understanding of the meaning of disability. They provide a basic introduction to the social model of disability and, in particular, the attitudinal, environmental, structural and language barriers that deny disabled people equal access to institutions and organizations. The following is a definition of a DET course (Gillespie-Sells & Campbell 1991:9):

> A DET course will enable participants to identify and address discriminatory forms of practice towards disabled people. Through training they will find ways to challenge the organisational behaviour which reinforces negatives myths and values and which prevents disabled people from gaining equality and achieving full participation in society.

There are predominantly two types of disability training in practice: disability awareness and disability equality. Basically:

1. awareness training tends to focus on individual impairment and often involves simulation exercises
2. equality training, on the other hand, explores the concept of the social model of disability and is provided by disabled trainers.

Disability equality training uses discussion-based methods for teaching and learning rather than simulation and is devised and delivered by disabled people. Simulation exercises have been criticized for a number of reasons. For instance, a sighted person wearing a blindfold for an hour or two will receive a very distorted and unrealistic understanding of disability (French 1996a). Nevertheless, this is a complex issue. In therapy practice, for instance, students do 'practice on each other'. However, this can have purposes other than to provide an apparent understanding of disability. For example, students may practice different crutch walking techniques on each other, not to understand what it feels like to have a broken leg, but simply to get practice in teaching crutch walking skills before beginning their work with patients.

Organizations are becoming increasingly aware of their role in providing 'customer care' for all their customers and clients. As Priestley (1999) points out, DET is now an established (albeit small) part of social work training courses in Britain. The Department of Health guidance on care management and assessment states that 'The most effective way of demonstrating the centrality of users' needs and wishes will be by consulting users and carers over the training programme and inviting them to contribute to the training itself' (Department of Health and Social Services Inspectorate & Scottish Office Social Work Services Group 1991:para. 106). Furthermore, the United Nations' standard rules on the equalization of opportunities for people with disabilities stipulates that disabled people's organizations should be involved in training development and that disabled people 'should be involved as teachers, instructors or advisers' (United Nations 1993:Rule 19.3). Awareness in Britain has been increased, in part, by the high profile of the Disability Discrimination Act (1995) and also by the awareness raising initiatives being put in place by leading and local disabled individuals and disability groups. Oliver & Barnes (1998:90) argue that the widespread use of DET as a radical new method of consciousness raising has played a role in intensifying 'the pressure for nothing less than the full inclusion of disabled people with comprehensive civil rights legislation as the main vehicle for its achievement'.

There is evidence to suggest that DET is not widely offered to health professionals on an in-service basis (Vernon et al 2001). Furthermore the research suggests that courses offered under the umbrella of DET differ in terms of their aims, who delivers them and how they are delivered. Disability equality training is not necessarily delivered by trainers who have been trained by organizations of disabled people. Also, some distance-learning packages which claim to offer DET are designed to raise awareness of impairment, though this strategy has been rejected by organizations of disabled people, and research evidence has repeatedly shown that such a strategy is ineffective in challenging social barriers (Vernon et al 2001).

◆ *Activity* 2.9

WHAT IS DISABILITY EQUALITY TRAINING?

This activity is based on information from a research project that investigated the provision of DET throughout Britain (Vernon et al 2001). Here we will give you a flavour of the views of disability equality trainers. As you read make a few notes of what you regard as the main points.

Purposes of training

The training, according to the trainers, is universal and is designed to improve both attitudes towards, and services for, disabled people. One trainer thought that the purpose of the training was 'To challenge misconceptions and break down barriers' (p. 13), while another said 'I think independence is a key word, to make people see that we can do things our way and by ourselves if we want to' (p. 14). Others recognized that attitude change tends to be slow and that the purpose of training is to 'plant seeds' of information.

There was some evidence to suggest that those who commission training do so for a variety of reasons. The role of the Disability Discrimination Act in serving as a carrot and, in some cases, a stick, is apparent. One participant said:

I found recently ... people are wanting their front line staff trained because of the DDA coming in. A lot of companies are panicking now and thinking, 'Where's the first point of contact that we're likely to be sued at?'

(p. 14)

This participant was critical of using DET in this way as it is geared towards the 'mechanics' of the Act rather than disability issues in a broader sense.

Training strategies

Disability trainers, whether orientated to equality or awareness, stressed the importance of the social model of disability. They also felt strongly that training should be as comfortable for the trainees as possible. One disability equality trainer recognized that attending a course can often be threatening for the participants: it was felt, for instance, that those receiving training should be helped to understand language use rather than, as one participant said, having it '... forced down their throats' (p. 14).

One disability awareness trainer saw the benefit of using simulation training methods. He stated that he specialized 'In making people blind for the afternoon, to show them how it feels' (p. 14). The majority of research participants, however, were very critical of the use of simulation exercises: one participant said that 'Any form of simulation exercise just trivialises disability' and another explained:

The only thing about doing these simulation techniques is ... that it gives people the opportunity to think, 'Oh, well I tried that' ... and it actually weakens the whole argument about looking at issues because you feel 'Well I've been there, I've done that, I've walked in your shoes' type of assumption.

(p. 15)

Target audiences

It was recognized by research participants that the effectiveness of the training depended on how it was delivered. While some organizations adopt a 'top-down' approach, others prefer one that is 'bottom-up'. Trainers argued that there has to be commitment from management if training is to result in anything practical and for it to influence policy change throughout the organizational culture. On many occasions the idea that training should be compulsory was raised. This was particularly in relation to medical staff: one participant thought that both doctors and psychologists should receive disability equality training early in their education and that refresher courses should be available later in their careers.

The issues raised in this report are complex. The participants are not simply addressing the development of knowledge and skills, but challenging and changing understandings of disability and professional policy, practice and provision. The following is taken from the recommendations of the report. You might find it helpful to compare these with the points you raised.

Control by disabled people

The overwhelming majority of research participants recognize that control by disabled people is fundamental to the development of DET. Disabled people should participate not only as trainers, but as trainers of the trainers, and they should also participate in the whole decision-making process of planning, organizing and evaluating DET. Such control and participation should be realized, not only through the democratic representation of organizations of disabled people, but also through a wide process of consultation.

Joined-up thinking

Mapping the provision of DET has led to the recommendation of 'joined-up' thinking both vertically and horizontally.

Vertical joined-up thinking refers to the need for all staff within an organization to receive training, from the front line staff to those at the senior management level. The report advises that there needs to be consistency in training vertically throughout the organization in order for policy change to be effective. Horizontal joined-up thinking refers to the need for organizations to work together to achieve consistency in training across all agencies. This applies to sectors working together, sharing best practice and recognizing the links between service provision and service providers.

Standard of training

There should be some system of recognition for trainers, to achieve the consistency recommended above. It was generally felt, however, that the development of a generic package is highly problematic and could disempower the grassroots participation of disabled trainers. At the very least, a standard package should be flexible enough to adapt to suit the audience. The following aspects of training packages were recommended by the overwhelming majority of the research participants:

1. Generic training should be a compulsory part of all staff induction packages.

2. Current staff may need retraining for up-to-date information.

3. Training should not be a 'one off'; it should be repeated and updated throughout employment.

4. Advanced training, with specific reference to the issues affecting that organization, should be available to all staff.

5. Advice for particular situations should be accessible within the organization on an ad hoc basis.

6. Training should include 'tailor-made' follow-up work. This could take on a work-based learning approach, whereby staff are asked to return to their places of employment and consider the issues with respect to their particular workplace. Trainers could then return at a later date to reiterate and assess the impact of the training.

Knowledge of disability

Experience of disability at a personal level is an essential requirement of being a trainer.

Central advice

Disability is complex, and both commonalties and diversities need to be recognized. Disabled people face a vast range of attitudinal, environmental and structural barriers and trainees cannot possibly be aware of everyone's needs from attending a training event. Advice needs to be available on an ad hoc basis for specific help in the form of a central advice bureau which is managed by disabled people.

Professional training

With participants' comments in mind, it is suggested, particularly for medical professionals who receive predominantly medical model training, that DET should form an integral part of their academic learning qualification.

Activity 2.10

WHAT ARE YOUR PROFESSIONAL DEVELOPMENT NEEDS?

Let us turn then to the therapy training you have undertaken or are currently undertaking. Examine the curriculum of your course and its relevance, or not, to working with disabled people. In the light of our previous discussions about DET, what skills and knowledge do you think are required and were these covered in the course curriculum? This activity may be difficult if you are just beginning your course. It will be useful, however, to focus on your expectations for professional development.

You might have considered some of the following issues:

- Is the individual model of disability predominant within your course?

- If so, what emphasis is given to the views of disabled people? Is the message of the course that the treatment of impairment can be appropriate if it is what disabled people want and if it fits in with their desired lifestyles?

- Does the course address therapist–client power relations? What emphasis is put on a relationship of equality?

- Is the social model covered within the course?

- If so, how? Is it central to the curriculum or an appendix? How much time in sessions is it given and is the tutor disabled? Is it addressed within the assignments and assessment of your course?

- Finally is the complex and disputed relationship between the two models examined within the course?

The question 'What is disability?' is like a stone dropped into a lake that creates ever increasing circles of questions. Our aim in dropping the stone here is to provide you with a basis for identifying and considering your own professional development needs. It is the basis too for you to develop your thinking about what you are looking for from this book.

CONCLUSION

Behind many of the debates in this chapter is the notion that there are two groups in society: disabled people and non-disabled people. Without denying the importance of this view of the social world in which we live, we would like to suggest an alternative way of thinking. Disability issues involve us all – the whole society. This argument can take many forms. There is, for instance, a numbers argument. In official statistics more than 1 in 10 of the UK population are disabled and more than 1 in 4 have direct experiences through family members (Giddens 2006). For us, however, there is a stronger argument. The social division between disabled people and non-disabled people is the one social divide that people cross daily through, for example, a car accident, contraction of a chronic illness or the deterioration of a physical condition. Furthermore, the longer we live the more likely it is that we will become impaired. Thus, the social treatment of disabled people is not simply a concern for people who are presently disabled. A non-disablist world is a vision for us all, not just one section of society.

Chapter 3

How did we get here?

In this chapter we will be considering the historical factors that have brought physiotherapists, occupational therapists and disabled people together in their present relationship. On the surface this association might seem obvious – disabled people have impairments which may need treating and therapists have the knowledge and skills that are required. Although this is one explanation, we hope to show, by outlining the history of disabled people as well as the history of the physiotherapy and occupational therapy professions, that social, economic and political factors are critically important. Since the formation of the Disabled People's Movement (see Ch. 2) disabled people have analysed and documented their history, including their experience of professional services. We believe that it is very important that therapists have some understanding of this history, and the role they have played within it, to understand and inform their current and future practice with disabled people. We hope that the content of this chapter will be useful in understanding therapy practice today. At the end of the chapter we will set an activity that asks you to reflect upon this issue.

THE DEVELOPMENT OF PHYSIOTHERAPY AND OCCUPATIONAL THERAPY IN THE EARLY YEARS

In this discussion we only need to turn the clock back about one hundred years because before that time the physiotherapy and occupational therapy professions did not exist. That having been said, physiotherapy developed from nursing and many techniques that are still used today – hydrotherapy, massage, manipulation, exercise therapy – date back to earlier centuries (Barclay 1994). Galen (129–216 AD), who was an eminent physician of his day, for instance, promoted exercise and treatment with water and was well aware of the impact of psychology (the 'passions of the soul') on health and illness. Specific people (usually of very low status) were employed to undertake these treatments. For example, 'rubber nurses' were employed by physicians in the 18th century to undertake massage (Kusukawa 2004).

Occupational therapy emerged as a profession in the USA in 1917 (Schwartz 2003). The first British occupational therapist started work in psychiatry in 1925 – a field that physiotherapists entered much later – and the first occupational therapy college opened in 1930 (Jay et al 1992). The early occupational therapists entered training with diplomas in arts and crafts. However, the concept of the therapeutic use of occupation dates back to Galen who advocated digging, fishing, ploughing and other activities to restore health (Macdonald 1976). Paterson (2002:4) states that:

> From the very earliest surviving manuscripts and throughout the ages, both in Eastern and in Western culture, we find reference to the belief that occupation in the form of exercise, work, recreation and amusements can both influence and be used to improve mental and physical health and well-being.

Occupational therapy has more recent roots in the mental asylums of the early 19th century that espoused a humanitarian ethos and where instructors were employed to encourage creative pursuits and recreational activities (Dunton 1957). As the 19th century progressed, however, the asylums became large, overcrowded and impersonal and the creative and recreational activities gave way to repetitive work with purely economic aims. Occupational therapy did not really emerge in Britain, however, until the Second World War. In 1937 there were just 37 registered occupational therapists in the whole of the UK (Jay et al 1992).

◆ *Activity 3.1*

THE DEVELOPMENT OF PHYSIOTHERAPY AND OCCUPATIONAL THERAPY IN THEIR WORK WITH DISABLED PEOPLE

Some people reading this book will have an excellent knowledge of recent British history whereas others will have a passing familiarity.

Whatever your situation, spend a few minutes thinking about the 20th century up until the end of the Second World War (1945). List any events and conditions that might have occurred to bring about and influence the association between disabled people and physiotherapists and occupational therapists. When you have done this write a few notes on:

- how far therapists benefited during this period in terms of their status and growth
- how far disabled people benefited in terms of their wellbeing and lifestyle.

Perhaps the first event that came to your mind when thinking about the early years of the 20th century in relation to disability was the First World War. This created a large number of disabled people, mostly young men, with a wide range of impairments including amputations, blindness and fractures. Many others experienced 'shell shock' – a condition we now describe as post-traumatic stress syndrome. It is well known that the First World War served as a catalyst for the expansion of the physiotherapy profession – or the Society of Trained Masseuses as it was called (Barclay 1994). Military hospitals and convalescent homes, both in Britain and overseas, were established, where physiotherapists were employed. This led to a considerable expansion in their numbers from 530 in 1911 to approximately 6000 in 1920 (Barclay 1994). The Shepherd's Bush Military Hospital in London, for example, was established in 1916 as an orthopaedic centre that employed both doctors and physiotherapists. It was the first centre specifically for the treatment of disabled adults (Resnick 2000). Many surgical procedures were undertaken and physiotherapists treated their patients with exercise, massage and electrotherapy. Handicraft instructors were also employed in the hospitals to teach and supervise crafts such as basketry and raffia work, both as a diversion and as a means of strengthening muscles and mobilizing joints following injury (Resnick 2000). The First World War also provided the impetus for the development of occupational therapy in the USA (Schwartz 2003).

Another factor you may have considered was the immense level of poverty in Britain at this time that led to a high incidence of impairment, especially among children in poor communities. These impairments included tuberculosis, rickets, polio and heart defects that were often caused by rheumatic fever. Medical examinations which were conducted to select young men for the Boer War (1899–1902) and the First World War

(1914–1918) uncovered an enormous amount of physical and sensory impairment, particularly among those from poor communities – 1 000 000 men were rejected for service on the grounds of poor health in the First World War (Barclay 1994). This led to greater medical surveillance of young people, initiated by government, in order that the nation should have a ready supply of fit young men to serve in the forces and to work in industry. In 1907, for example, annual medical inspection of all school children was introduced.

The high level of poverty and increasing concern about the nation's health, gave much scope for the development of physiotherapy. In the 1930s, for example, physiotherapists treated large numbers of children with rickets (caused by lack of vitamin D) with ultraviolet radiation. Betty Duke, who practised physiotherapy in the 1930s, recalled treating

> ... little tiny children, just with their nappies on, sitting cross-legged on the floor around these lamps ... They were there to get some sunlight because Camden Town was full of slums. (Oxlade & French 2005:26)

Physiotherapists were also involved in the keep-fit movement of the 1930s which was promoted by government to improve public health during the economic depression and high unemployment of the inter-war years (Barclay 1994).

A further factor that led to the 'coming together' of disabled people and physiotherapists and occupational therapists at this time was the rise in the eugenics movement which sought to 'improve' the human race by controlling reproduction by, for instance, segregation, sterilization and the prevention of marriage and emigration (Snyder & Mitchell 2006). Snyder & Mitchell propose that the eugenics movement lies at the root of all professions concerned with disability. They state (2006:524–625):

> ... an ideological practice cloaked in the empiricism of scientific research ... the eugenics movement gave birth to the contemporary focus of nearly every social and therapeutic discipline that attempts to treat and manage disabled people today: physical therapy, occupational therapy, social work, genetics, genetic counseling, special education and community and applied psychology.

Doctors were at the forefront of this movement and had top positions in the Nazi concentration camps where they experimented upon and murdered hundreds of thousands of disabled people (Evans 2004). In view of this history it is not surprising that the relationship between disabled people and medical professionals is uneasy, especially as eugenic ideals are still expressed in prenatal screening, abortion, genetic counselling and genetic engineering (Kerr & Shakespeare 2002, Parens & Asch 2000).

The eugenics movement, as well as other influences such as changes in working practices since the Industrial Revolution, led to a greater number of disabled people being incarcerated in various institutions run by the state and charities (Borsay 2005). This was paralleled by an increase in the number of therapists working in hospitals, schools for physically disabled children and psychiatric and mental handicap asylums. It can be seen that the growth and development of physiotherapy and occupational therapy, and indeed all the health professions, has gone hand in hand with government policy.

It is clear that the physiotherapy profession in particular benefited during this period and became stronger and more secure. Physiotherapists worked within the infrastructure established by government in the First World War to treat badly injured service men. The services of physiotherapists were actively sought leading to increased prestige and rising numbers. The First World War enabled various medical specialties to develop, particularly orthopaedics, which led to the employment of still more physiotherapists and a rising number of occupational therapists.

Following the First World War it was in the interest of those who had worked within the military hospitals and convalescent homes to turn their attention to other disabled people and to use their facilities in a different way (Borsay 2005). As Bourke (1996:51) rather cynically puts it: '... the war time economy created an army of people whose livelihood was dependent upon maintaining a supply of cripples.' Resources were largely diverted to physically disabled children. In 1919 the Central Council for the Care of Cripples, which had representation from the medical profession, the state and the voluntary sector, was formed as a co-ordinating body. By 1925 there was institutional provision and after-care services for over 100 000 physically disabled children, many of whom were segregated for ten or more years and were subjected to hours of therapy and repeated surgical procedures (Borsay 2005). Later the hospitals were full of children who contracted poliomyelitis, in the epidemics of the 1940s and 1950s, many of whom spent years in hospital (Oswin 1971). The harshness of this regime is illustrated in the following quotations from two people who were hospitalized and treated for cerebral palsy and poliomyelitis when they were children:

> I was in hospital for five years and my mum used to visit me every week but she wasn't allowed into the ward, not once in all that time. She just looked in through the window in the ward door and waved to me like all the other parents. That was really upsetting,

much more upsetting than if we'd had proper visits. She used to leave me presents to have when she had gone home but of course it wasn't like seeing her properly. All year we looked forward to the garden fete in the summer so then we could be with our mums properly for an hour or so.

(Humphries & Gordon 1992:73)

From the age of five until I was thirteen I was encased in a plaster cast rather like an Egyptian mummy in the children's ward at the Royal Sea Bathing Hospital in Margate. Whenever the little girl in the bed next to me wanted to play 'dollies' I undid the straps that were meant to keep my arms still and joined in with the game. But if the nurse ever saw us, and she mostly did, she thundered down the ward, yelled at me, put me back in my little coffin and tied my hands and arms down with bandages to the side of the bed really tight … they would quite often wheel me, bed and all, into the cold, wet bathroom as a punishment. And I had to cry myself to sleep to the sound of the dripping tap.

(Humphries & Gordon 1992:81)

After the First World War doctors also turned their attention to the treatment of fractures and industrial injuries. Factory owners and mining companies would sometimes establish their own facilities where injured workers could be treated and returned to work as soon as possible. Sanatoriums for the treatment of tuberculosis was another area of medical growth at this time (Barclay 1994). All of these developments provided fertile ground for the expansion and development of both physiotherapy and occupational therapy.

The Second World War saw another expansion of these professions. The injuries people incurred during the Second World War tended to be multiple, which required teams of specialist doctors and therapists in their treatment. This led to a huge expansion of rehabilitation not just for people injured in war but also for disabled civilians. During the first half of 1945 for example, 30 000 people were being rehabilitated, a third of them as in-patients (Borsay 2005). The Second World War also saw the development of neurology as a medical specialty. Twelve dedicated units for spinal cord injuries were established at this time, including Stoke Mandeville that opened in 1944 (Barclay 1994). These units provided new openings and opportunities for physiotherapists and occupational therapists to specialize. During the Second World War the physiotherapy profession expanded by a fifth, from approximately 12 000 members in 1940 to 15 000 members in 1945 (Barclay 1994). The occupational therapy profession grew more slowly and by 1974 had 5783 members (Jay et al 1992) The Second World War did, however, provide a major impetus for its development (Macdonald 1976). It was not until the Second World War that occupational therapists became widely involved in treating patients with physical impairments, and by the 1950s attention was being paid to 'daily living skills' rather than simply the strengthening of muscles and the mobilization of joints (Schwartz 2003).

It would appear on the surface that disabled people benefited just as much as therapists from these developments, but a closer inspection highlights considerable problems for disabled people as well as definite gains – the survival rate following spinal cord injury, for instance, rose dramatically after the Second World War with the establishment of special units. It is important to realize, however, that therapists and other medical personnel were working within a government infrastructure that existed to serve the interests of the state. During the First World War, for example, the aim of medical personnel was to send men back to the front line where they had a high chance of being killed. The medical fraternity was also involved in identifying and exposing those who were thought to be malingering and screening out all but the most deserving cases from the provision of a war pension (Bourke 1996). The aims of medical staff and patients were, therefore, often completely opposed (Cooter 2004).

The rehabilitation of wounded people during the First and Second World Wars was intimately related to paid work and production, that were seen by the state to legitimize the resources they were putting into it. Resnick (2000:192), talking of the First World War, states that '… government policy towards disabled soldiers was intended to make these men healthy citizens for the benefit of post-war reconstruction.' At the Shepherd's Bush Military Hospital, for example, not only did the men undertake physiotherapy and handicrafts to improve their injuries and psychological state, but in the 'curative workshops' they were involved in furniture making, upholstery, car maintenance, tailoring, fretwork and photography to raise income. They also made and repaired medical equipment, such as splints, thereby benefiting the medical service directly. All of this was done without remuneration and there is evidence than many men resented the work and refused to do it (Resnick 2000). Sociologists such as Freidson (1970) assert that the medical profession is an 'agent of the state' which functions to maintain social order within society. According to Cooter (2004) the purpose of rehabilitation was, in part, to avoid social unrest among large groups of disaffected men.

Physiotherapists and occupational therapists who were involved in rehabilitation at this time undoubtedly helped some disabled people but they would have been working in opposition to others. Turner (2002) states that occupational therapy following the Second World War was vital in getting people back to work. Rehabilitation was, however, usually denied to people with progressive conditions or where there was little hope of improvement. As Borsay (2005:61) states:

> … their social right to rehabilitation under the NHS was impeded by the construction of impairment as a pathology remediable through the performance of a specific set of 'technical activities'. With this mindset in place, the majority of disabled people with static or deteriorating conditions were excluded from rehabilitation services that differently conceived could have supported the achievement of personal autonomy within particular social contexts.

People disabled by war were given priority over those born disabled or disabled by disease or industrial accidents. There was a transfer of resources, not just in terms of medical staff, but also in terms of accommodation such as workshops and homes. People disabled by war were young, fit and often well educated and thus had more political influence than civilian disabled people. First World War veterans, for example, succeeded in their campaign for free, lightweight, metal artificial limbs, rather than the cumbersome wooden ones, whereas no artificial limbs of any kind were provided for civilian disabled people until after the Second World War (Bourke 1996). Charities specifically for people disabled by war were set up which tended to be wealthier than those for other disabled people. The following quotation from a physiotherapist who was born visually impaired and who trained alongside those who had been blinded in the Second World War, and were assisted by the charity St Dunstan's, illustrates this point:

> They went under the banner of St Dunstan's which suggested somebody who had given his sight for his country, whereas somebody like myself, who had been born partially sighted – well OK hard luck! … The St Dunstan's students had this lovely place in Park Crescent where they were waited on by VADs, while we had a crummy hostel in New Barnet with a dreadful landlady who reported everything we did. So we were a bit antagonistic and jealous I suppose.
>
> (French 2001:56)

War-blinded physiotherapists were assisted by St Dunstan's throughout their careers, as a physiotherapist explains:

> Their help was very practical. All of my working life, until a couple of years ago, there was a sighted physio who did nothing but look

after the chaps' interests … You could ring him up and say, 'my machine's broken down' and he'd come and sort it out. He also organised our annual congress for us and visited us every two or three months. He was someone to lean on for the practical side of things.

(French 2001:57)

Families were often held responsible for impairments that occurred in peace time and workers were frequently blamed for the industrial injuries they incurred. In contrast, people who were disabled by war were thought to be the nation's responsibility, although their privileged position over other disabled people tended to be short lived (Bourke 1996). Thus, although people who were disabled by war may have been helped by charities and medical personnel, such as physiotherapists and occupational therapists, it created inequalities among disabled people and led, in some instances, to large numbers of disabled people becoming more disadvantaged than they had previously been (Bourke 1996).

During the first half of the 20th century many disabled people lived in institutions and their lives were increasingly medicalized. This tendency started in the 19th century when the state made doctors responsible for numerous decisions about disabled people's lives including who was eligible for Poor Law relief, who needed special education and who should be diagnosed as insane (Borsay 2005). Although the majority of disabled people have always lived in the community, the number living in institutions rose substantially and many became segregated, self-contained communities. Chailey Heritage which was opened in 1903, for example, provided hospital treatment, education and vocational training. It was also common practice for the inhabitants of institutions to be heavily involved in running them by undertaking such tasks as gardening, laundering, farming, cleaning and caring for less able residents. This was done with little or no remuneration and usually under an abusive regime (Potts & Fido 1991). I (Sally) spent my early years in Lingfield, a village in Surrey, where there was a large 'colony' for people with epilepsy. This was a self-contained, segregated community with its own farm, laundry, workshops and school.

Disability was perceived by the state and by the medical profession and therapists as being a problem located within the individual. This was harmful to disabled people as it placed the emphasis on changing *them* rather than on adjusting the physical and social environment to accommodate their needs. As noted above, children who were undernourished were treated with artificial sunlight by physiotherapists rather than providing them with a more nutritious diet or improved living conditions. Similarly, many disabled children continued to spend years in hospital having surgery and therapy while little attention was paid to an environment beset with barriers (Borsay 2005).

It is clear that, as physiotherapists and occupational therapists gained in strength and status during the first half of the 20th century, little attention was paid to the lifestyles or wellbeing of disabled people. The increasing segregation and the strong influence of the medical profession in defining disability led to disabled people becoming less visible in the community and being regarded as sick and in need of 'special' care, though, in effect, little care or treatment was provided (Ryan & Thomas 1990). Medical professionals increasingly had control over the lives of large numbers of disabled people and the help they received was increasingly 'professionalized'. Undoubtedly some disabled people gained by the expansion of medical services but many others suffered serious injustices and abuse at the hands of those who sought to cure them, 'normalize' them or remove them from mainstream society. Disabled people are highly critical of the policies and practices that led to and maintained their marginalization and oppression, and have recently been speaking out about their experiences (see French et al 2006, Humphries & Gordon 1992, Potts & Fido 1991).

THE WELFARE STATE

In 1942 the Beveridge Report was published, which resulted from the work of a committee chaired by Sir William Beveridge. The Beveridge Report led to the establishment of the welfare state through a raft of social legislation aimed at improving the living conditions of the British population. Beveridge thought that the welfare state would put an end to what he referred to as the 'five giants'. These are shown in Box 3.1.

Box 3.1

1. Want – the welfare state would provide an adequate income.
2. Disease – the welfare state would provide access to health care.
3. Ignorance – the welfare state would provide access to educational opportunities.
4. Squalor – the welfare state would provide adequate housing.
5. Idleness – the welfare state would provide gainful employment.

Beveridge believed that these welfare reforms would provide care for everyone 'from cradle to grave' (Timmins 2001).

The founding principles of the welfare state were universalism (certain rights, like the right to a home, should apply to everyone), statism (that the state should intervene in important areas of life such as health care and housing), egalitarianism (that there should be equal opportunities), nationalism (that industries such as gas and water should be owned by the state so that everyone would have access to necessities) and the redistribution of wealth through taxation (Lovell & Cordeaux 1999). The Acts shown in Box 3.2 were passed over a number of years in an attempt to achieve these aims.

Box 3.2

- 1944 Education Act
- 1945 Family Allowance Act
- 1946 National Insurance Act
- 1946 National Insurance (industrial injuries) Act
- 1946 National Health Service Act
- 1947 Town and Country Planning Act
- 1947 New Towns Act
- 1948 National Assistance Act
- 1948 Children Act
- 1949 Housing Act

(From Lovell & Cordeaux 1999, with permission from Edward Arnold (Publishers) Ltd)

The centrepiece of the plan was a state-run system of compulsory insurance. Workers would contribute to National Insurance through their pay packet. This would build up a fund to pay benefits to sick, injured and unemployed people. The scheme would also pay pensions at the end of a working life.

For those who did not contribute to National Insurance, and therefore fell outside the scheme, there was a second tier of welfare provision, National Assistance, which was means tested. The welfare state was said to provide universal access to secondary education and the health service that were financed through taxation and were free at the point of delivery. Beveridge thought that the health service would become cheaper as people's health improved. Some of the ideas put forward in the Beveridge Report were modified before they became legislation and other modifications occurred during the first few years of the welfare state. For example, payment for spectacles and prescription fees were implemented in 1949 (Timmins 2001).

Health care was much more visible than social care and was said to be the 'jewel in the crown' of the welfare reforms. Social care was not nearly so well thought through or so well financed and far more resources went into 'cure' than into 'care'. When setting up the NHS the government had to negotiate with the powerful medical profession. The result of this was a service with three arms (Ham 1999) as shown in Box 3.3.

Box 3.3

1. The hospital and specialist medical services
This consumed most of the resources. There was, however, a hierarchy of hospitals with the acute hospitals and teaching hospitals being well funded whereas others, such as geriatric hospitals and the asylums for people with learning difficulties and mental health problems, became 'backwaters'.

2. Family practitioner services
These included services by GPs, dentists and ophthalmic opticians.

3. Local authority services
These included district nurses, health visitors, mental health services and services for disabled people.

Part of the National Assistance Act (1948) established welfare departments in local authorities, putting a duty on them to provide accommodation for old, disabled and homeless people and to promote the welfare of disabled people. They had few powers to support people at home and it was assumed that much could be left to voluntary services and the family. The NHS did, however, inherit some elements of social care such as the mental handicap asylums and some institutions for old people (Timmins 2001). These institutions had an appalling history of abuse and neglect that continued under the NHS (Ryan & Thomas 1990). As Welshman (2006:36) states:

> ... the powerful sociological critique of institutional care had by the late 1960s been augmented by evidence of scandals relating to ill-treatment, stealing and indifference on the part of staff.

The establishment of the welfare state, particularly the NHS, provided another spur for the development of occupational therapy and physiotherapy (Schwartz 2003). Most occupational therapists and physiotherapists were employed within the NHS in a wide range of medical specialties (Barclay 1994, Schwartz 2003). Occupational therapists were also gradually employed within the community under the control of local authorities. This increased with the passing of the Chronically Sick and Disabled Persons Act (1970) that was the first welfare legislation specifically focused on disabled people. It made mandatory the provision of various services for disabled people in the community including equipment and home adaptations (Schwartz 2003). The legislation was, however, weak and centred on the individual rather than on the environment. It also confirmed the erroneous connection between disability and chronic sickness which influenced the development of future services.

Activity 3.2

LIVING IN A GERIATRIC WARD

Read the following extract about Miss Turner, a disabled person in a long-stay geriatric hospital, and then consider the questions at the end.

As a physiotherapy student in 1969, I (Sally) worked on a female long-stay geriatric ward in a large general hospital in North London. It had a row of beds down either side and the nursing station at the top. The ward, which was very short-staffed, was dirty and smelt of urine. Bits of food crunched under foot. The patients did not get dressed; some wandered about in their night clothes while others lay in bed or lolled in their chairs. Many patients were demented – I remember Annie who loved to play with water and often made a terrible mess.

Amidst this scene of desolation and mayhem was Miss Turner. Miss Turner was a small woman in her forties with advanced multiple sclerosis. This ward had been her 'home' for many years – and would almost certainly be her last. As students we treated Miss Turner twice a day by stretching the contractures in her legs. She seemed to enjoy our company but often resisted the treatment (which was painful) but it took place nonetheless. She constantly complained that Annie, and some of the other patients, stole her belongings. Miss Turner had a manual typewriter and would occupy herself as best she could by writing, but her work would often disappear – nobody seemed interested in this or in what she was writing about. She did not talk about her life and she never divulged her first name. Our clinical supervisor, who was meticulous in teaching us physiotherapy techniques, did not seem interested in Miss Turner as a person with a past.

- What factors could have led to a young woman like Miss Turner being placed in a long-term geriatric ward?
- Why was so little notice taken of Miss Turner as a person?
- Should physiotherapy have been such a priority when Miss Turner's life was so impoverished?
- How far do you consider that the relationship between Miss Turner and the physiotherapists was equal?
- Explain some of the social, economic and political factors which could have brought Miss Turner and the physiotherapists together in this particular context.

I do not remember learning anything about Miss Turner's social situation but it is likely that she had nobody to assist her in the community and lived on this ward because there was nowhere else for her to go. This situation was not unusual for young disabled people at this time. Large numbers lived in institutions including homes run by local authorities (who were responsible for providing them with accommodation under the 1948 National Assistance Act), charities (such as Leonard Cheshire) and NHS geriatric and general wards (Oliver 1983). Talking of young disabled people in the 1960s, Battye (1966:14) states that '… sooner or later he will find himself a patient in the chronic ward of a long-stay hospital surrounded by the old, the incontinent and the dying.' As noted above, little resources were put into community or long-term care. In response to the Chronically Sick and Disabled Person's Act (1970), NHS institutions specifically for younger disabled people were built in order to remove them from hospital wards, particularly geriatric wards. As Shearer (1974:62) states:

> The government has been urging an increase in younger chronic sick units on its hospital boards since 1968 when a survey found that half the 4200 or so severely disabled people being catered for by the NHS were on geriatric wards … Another 1300 were on general hospital wards.

Forty-one 'Young Chronic Sick Units' were established by 1973 but their progress was slowed down by consumer resistance as disabled people were beginning to see the possibility of a brighter future for themselves outside residential care (Oliver 1983).

It is likely that little notice was taken of Miss Turner as a person because she was regarded as a patient and, furthermore, was within a medical specialty (geriatrics) where patients were not highly valued. The staff who came into contact with Miss Turner had specific roles to perform (mostly of a biomedical nature) and would have concentrated on those roles rather than socializing with Miss Turner or finding out about her life.

Miss Turner had physiotherapy twice a day but very little else. The physiotherapy may have helped to prevent the contractures in her legs getting worse but it is likely that the treatment she received was more for the benefit of the students than herself. Miss Turner lived in a hospital and her life was utterly medicalized so physiotherapy would have seemed the 'natural' thing to do rather than, for instance, arranging interesting trips outside the hospital or providing Miss Turner with equipment or a personal helper. As noted above rehabilitation was generally restricted at this time to young people whose conditions were likely to improve or at least not deteriorate while others, like Miss Turner, were either left with their families or abandoned in long-stay institutions (Borsay 2005).

The relationship between Miss Turner and the physiotherapists (even though they were mostly students) was highly unequal. Miss Turner was given treatment whether she wanted it or not and at times that suited the therapists. It was assumed that the therapists were the experts regarding Miss Turner's condition and, although she would have lived with multiple sclerosis for many years, her opinions were never sought and her experience was not valued.

It is likely that Miss Turner had few resources as disabled people then, as now, were among the poorest in society (Barnes 1991). Unemployment among disabled people was very high so most would not have paid into the National Insurance scheme. Care in the community (in the absence of a family that was willing and able to cope) was virtually non-existent at this time (Morris 1993a) and there was little in the way of adapted housing available – the Housing Act and New Towns Act did not take disabled people's access needs into account. Disabled people were not a high priority of the NHS, or other areas of government policy, and very limited resources were put towards their health and wellbeing – though some provision for wheelchairs and mobility aids was made. It can be seen that the welfare state did not provide equally for all of its citizens and many groups such as disabled people and old people were poorly served. Miss Turner's hospitalization can also be seen in the context of the history of the institutionalization of disabled people that stretches over the course of the 20th century and beyond (Borsay 2005).

Although we have chosen to focus on Miss Turner in this account, the lives of Annie and the other people on the ward were equally as shocking and in need of improvement, as highlighted by Townsend in his book *The Last Refuge* (1962).

◆ *Activity* 3.3

LIVING IN A RESIDENTIAL SCHOOL

Read the following extract about a special school for disabled children, where I (Sally) worked in my teenage years. Then answer the questions at the end.

From 1965 until 1967 I worked as an assistant housemother in a residential school for children with cerebral palsy which was run by the Spastics Society (now SCOPE). I was 16 when I started and came straight from school. There were fourteen other childcare workers employed, some of whom were qualified in child care, and 55 children with severe physical disabilities and mild learning difficulties. The school was situated in an old manor house at the end of a long, winding drive with woods either side. The nearest town was seven miles away. Visiting days were very restricted and the school was difficult to reach without a car. Some of the children lived far away and only went home at holiday times. Those without parents who could care for them were placed in long-stay children's hospitals during the holidays.

Four physiotherapists were employed at the school as well as a part-time speech and language therapist. The children received therapy several times a week and it was our job, as care assistants, to collect them from their classrooms, prepare them for therapy and then take them back. There was no liaison between the teachers and the therapists but therapy was always given priority. The physiotherapy department was well equipped and there was a good-sized hydrotherapy pool which the children also used for recreational activities some weekends. I do not remember the physiotherapists teaching me or the other care workers anything about what they were doing – although we often watched. The speech and language therapist was more forthcoming and would sometimes spend a few minutes explaining what she hoped to achieve. Many of the children were profoundly deaf but we were not given any tuition in sign language or any other form of communication with them although specialist teachers were employed.

There were no electric wheelchairs at the school and most of the children were too impaired to walk or to move about unaided in manual wheelchairs. Great emphasis was placed on preventing deformities and children would have their feet strapped into the 'correct' position and their knees held apart with wooden wedges most of the time. The hydrotherapy pool gave some children freedom of movement and others could ride tricycles when their feet and hands were securely strapped into place. At the weekends we ventured to the top of the drive, each pushing two wheelchairs, where there was a sweet shop. Once in a while we went to the sea and we also had picnics in the woods. We were very isolated from the community although some weekends boys from a nearby public school came to play with the children.

- How similar or dissimilar do you find the situation of the children in this special school to that of Miss Turner?
- What are your thoughts and feelings about the therapy that the disabled children received?
- Why were the children in this segregated, special school?

It is likely that you found the lives of the children at this school rather less bleak than that of Miss Turner and the other patients on the geriatric ward. The school was well staffed, some outings were arranged and there was a little time to give the children individual attention.

However, the children were very isolated and rarely saw their families. Many of the people looking after them were very young, totally untrained and often unsupervised.

The children received a great deal of physiotherapy – four physiotherapists for 55 children is a high ratio. You may have felt that this overmedicalized their lives and that therapy was given too high a priority when compared with leisure time and education. You may also have felt that the philosophy of restricting movement in order to prevent deformity was too confining or even abusive. As a disabled person, quoted by Davies (1992:37), said:

> Looking back from the age of nine to sixteen the primary aim of that school was to 'therup' me. It had nothing to do with education really.

The physiotherapists did not communicate greatly with the teaching staff or care staff and the staff, as a whole, did not work as a team. The therapists worked largely within a medical model philosophy and focused on their own particular areas of expertise. In this way the situation of the children was highly medicalized and similar to that of Miss Turner. As with Miss Turner, this was a time of few resources in the community for disabled people or their families and limited inclusion for disabled children in mainstream schools (Hurt 1988).

Oswin (1971) compared the lives of the children in this particular school with those of children living in long-stay hospital wards and found much to recommend the school. This was in terms of the high staff/child ratio, staff continuity, the presence of toys, the lack of queuing, living in more than one room and the opportunity for some individual attention. She was also positive about the therapy the children received. Although this school would now fall far short of acceptable childcare practice, the children were considerably better off than the many who were housed in long-stay hospitals. Special schools tended to be selective and Oswin (1971) noted that many hospitalized children were never offered a place in a special school. Furthermore, until the 1970 Education Act children who were labelled as having severe learning difficulties were not entitled to an education and the Children Act (1948) did not cover disabled children (Oswin 1971).

The children in this school, as well as Miss Turner, represent the lives of thousands of disabled people at this time who were living with few resources in segregated institutions. The welfare state focused primarily on the needs of the 'normal' nuclear family – an able-bodied man with his wife and children – and many groups, such as disabled people, lone parents and those from ethnic minorities were left on the margins of society with few provisions being made for them (Lewis 1998).

When discussing the experiences of disabled people from a historical perspective, such as Miss Turner and the children in the special residential school, it is important to realize that the issues have not been 'laid to rest'. Many of the people who went through these experiences are still alive, and may well bear the scars. Furthermore there is much that needs to be done before we can claim that disabled people are equal citizens or that they no longer live in segregated institutions.

RESTRUCTURING THE WELFARE STATE

By the time that Margaret Thatcher was elected as prime minister of the Conservative Party in 1979, the welfare state was under severe strain due to a number of diverse factors including:

- an ageing population
- rising unemployment
- recession and high inflation
- shrinkage of the manufacturing industry and the economy generally
- more separation, divorce and lone parents – the welfare state was dependent on the existence of the conventional nuclear family
- more demands for health and social care.

The welfare state was also challenged by many new social movements, for example the Women's Movement, the Black Power Movement and the Disabled People's Movement, who had not been treated equally and were demanding full citizenship rights (Lewis 1998). This led, in the 1970s, to the passing of various Acts including the Sex Discrimination Act (1975) and the Race Relations Act (1976) which made it less acceptable to discriminate against women and people from ethnic minorities in terms, for example, of housing and health and social care. The passing of the Disability Discrimination Act took far longer to achieve and did not reach the statute book until 1995.

A radical new way of thinking, which came to be known as the New Right or Thatcherism emerged in the 1980s. All areas of public spending were radically re-organized and state involvement in welfare was reduced: tenants, for example, had the right to buy their council houses and head teachers managed their own budgets. There was a legislative attack on trade unions in order to reduce their power and there were many restrictions placed on local authorities who were compelled to sell council houses and to put their services (such as the provision of accommodation for old and disabled people) out to competitive tendering (Langan 1998).

New Right's diagnosis of the problem of the welfare state was that public expenditure had been allowed to grow unchecked. Old virtues of self-help and thrift were espoused rather than relying on the 'nanny state'. Central and local government, as well as professionals, were seen as monopolies that rigidly imposed particular services on people, and wasted resources as there was no competition to keep them in check. The roles and expectations of welfare recipients were also challenged, with emphasis being placed on responsibility and individual autonomy rather than deference and dependency within a paternalistic system. This can be summarized under a number of principles that the New Right upheld (from Lovell & Cordeaux 1999:175–176):

- *Decentralization:* the state should have a minimal role in welfare provision.
- *Privatization:* private companies should own, organize and deliver services.
- *Self-help:* people should help themselves and help each other in the community.
- *Competition:* services should compete against each other as a means of raising standards and increasing efficiency.
- *Freedom of choice:* clients should have choice over which services they receive. This would be encouraged by competition and the reduction of professional and state monopoly.
- *Enterprise:* people should be encouraged to be innovative and creative in the services they provide.
- *Individualism:* people should be responsible for their own needs including their own care.

The New Right dealt with the problem as they saw it by introducing ideas from the commercial world. A new kind of management was required which would use business principles to reduce cost and increase efficiency. Such managerialism, it was hoped, would also serve to break down professional control and modify the power of the trade unions. Competition was introduced into the public sector in the belief that it would keep quality up and costs down. Shifts in language accompanied these changes: patients, clients and passengers, for example, became customers, which implied that they had greater choice and control. The discourse was that patients and clients would have more choice although this was disputed by many, including Walmsley (2006a:83), who states that 'The rhetoric of choice has been extensively deployed to justify this marketisation though … the link between consumer preference and the service provided is often hard to discern'.

In 1989 two white papers were published which formed the basis of the NHS and Community Care Act (1990). The white paper 'Working for Patients' (Department of Health 1989b) dealt with the NHS and set out ways in which competition could be introduced in the form of what is known as an 'internal' or 'quasi' market. District health authorities could 'shop around' among hospitals, rather than being restricted to their own. This created competition among a wide range of NHS and private hospitals. GPs managed their own budgets and had more choice regarding the services they could provide. Self-governing 'trust' hospitals were also formed which were outside the control of district health authorities. In time, community health services and ambulance services also became trusts (Butler & Calnan 1999). Services such as laundering, refuse collection, catering and cleaning were put out to competitive tendering and hospitals were encouraged to raise their own resources by, for example, opening flower shops, hairdressers and food outlets on their premises (Jones 2000). As Jones (2000:181) states:

> ... the Government's plan for the Health Service, as for other services, involved bringing in the efficiency and competition of the business world, and ultimately breaking up what was seen as a state monopoly in the hands of professional vested interests.

The white paper 'Caring for People' (Department of Health 1989a) was concerned with services in the community and how market principles would apply there. Before 1990 social service departments both planned and delivered care, they employed their own staff and supplied a limited range of services for their clients. Under the NHS and Community Care Act (1990), however, social service departments became purchasers rather than providers, with their role being to assess the needs of clients and issue contracts to others who would supply the services. This division was known as the purchaser–provider split. Those who wished to provide the services were in competition with each other and were obliged to bid for contracts. This resulted in what is referred to as a 'mixed economy of welfare' involving state, voluntary and private providers of services. Under this legislation clients are allocated a 'care manager' (a professional such as a social worker or occupational therapist) who assesses them and organizes 'packages of care' from a variety of statutory, private and voluntary organizations (Twigg 1998). A major drive of the NHS and Community Care Act (1990) was to close down large institutions, for example psychiatric and mental handicap hospitals, and provide care in the community. In 1990 there were still 32700 beds in mental handicap hospitals (Walmsley 2006a).

The NHS and Community Care Act (1990) made it mandatory to involve users in the planning and delivery of services and various charters were drawn up, for example the Patients' Charter, which were designed to give users more voice though they carry no legal status.

Activity 3.4

THE IMPACT OF NEW RIGHT POLICIES ON DISABLED PEOPLE AND THERAPISTS

Think about the changes that were brought into the area of health and social care during the Conservative Governments of 1979–1997.

- In what ways might these changes have benefited disabled people?
- In what ways might these changes have benefited physiotherapists and occupational therapists working with disabled people?
- Why were many people sceptical about the benefits of these changes in the lives of disabled people?

It was thought by many people that these changes would go some way to weakening the monopoly of both the state and professionals thereby providing disabled people with a greater range and choice of services. It was also envisaged that the 'care manager' would have an overview of the disabled person's needs and would work within a 'needs-led' rather than a 'resource-led' framework.

The possible benefits for physiotherapists and occupational therapists was that they would be working with disabled people in a relationship of greater equality where they could provide more flexible and creative services. This was particularly so in the social services where occupational therapists were employed. On the other hand, such changes posed a threat to therapists who feared a reduction of power and control if disabled people had more choice and more influences in the services they received. The NHS and Community Care Act (1990) provided new openings for occupational therapists (as care managers within social services) and for physiotherapists working in the community.

Some people were pessimistic about the changes that the NHS and Community Care Act (1990) would bring based upon the beliefs outlined in Box 3.4.

Box 3.4

- Lack of resources was the main problem and this would not be solved by the introduction of market forces into health and social care.
- Money would be wasted setting up new services and new administrative systems.
- Care work would be pushed onto unpaid carers – especially women.
- Employers of low-paid staff who were in competition would undercut each other reducing wages still further and that would adversely affect services.
- Charters would not be effective as they are not legal documents.
- Changes would not be based on clients' rights but on a desire to save money.

The image of the consumer exercising free choice in health and social care was also viewed as problematic due to the points outlined in Box 3.5.

Box 3.5

- An imbalance of power between those who provide the care and those who receive it.
- Finite and limited resources. More customers does not equal more money, as it does in a free market, and customers can be a cost rather than a source of income. Distribution of resources is an act of political will where the interests of individual consumers are juggled against the interests of the community as a whole.
- The purchasers of services have choice rather than the actual users – for example care managers and GPs. They have been termed 'proxy customers' and are usually public sector employees.
- Consumerism risks producing social inequalities by focusing on the individual and ignoring wider social factors.
- People may not want to be consumers. The choices may be too difficult at times of vulnerability where issues such as trust may be more important.

As these policies came into effect, disabled people found that their ideas of independent living in the community clashed with those of social service managers and professionals who focused on basic care – bathing, dressing and so on. Furthermore, assessments were geared to available resources rather than being 'needs led'. Over time 'packages of care' became more restrictive with tighter eligibility criteria and means testing. The emphasis was firmly on 'care' rather than 'quality of life' with few choices and little control. Furthermore, large charities, such as Leonard Cheshire, had the advantage when it came to bidding against smaller organizations, including those that were run by disabled people themselves, with the danger of monopoly and stifling innovation (Walmsley 2006a). The unequal power relationship between disabled people and professionals, not least because professionals are the gatekeepers of services, did not fundamentally change with this legislation but, rather, became obscured by notions of consultation and user involvement (French & Swain in press).

Some changes which disabled people regard as positive did, however, evolve from the NHS and Community Care Act (1990). The Direct Payment Act (1996), for example, enables local authorities to assess disabled people for a direct payment that they can spend on their own needs, including the services of care workers. This effectively gives disabled people the status of employers. The payment made is given following an assessment by a professional, and the disabled person may be monitored but, nonetheless, many disabled people find direct payments give them more control over their lives than when they rely on statutory and voluntary services. This is illustrated in the following quotations:

> With social service home care I felt that they came in, 'did me' and then went off and 'did' someone else. I was beholden to them. With direct payment I'm the boss and the employee has a different approach to me as I'm paying them rather than someone sending them to help a hopeless person.
>
> (Dawson 2000:19)

> Employing my own personal assistant has given me the freedom to fulfil the type of lifestyle I wish to follow. I can go where I want when I want. I am in total control of making all the choices in my life. I feel I am much more my own person once again able to put all my abilities to some useful purpose.
>
> (Oliver & Zarb 1992:9)

Despite the popularity of direct payments there are still problems of access for some groups, for example people from ethnic minorities and people with learning difficulties, and various complex concerns such as the responsibility of being an employer, the possibility of exploitation and coping with the complex relationship between a disabled person and a personal assistant (Leece & Bornat 2006).

Activity *3.5*

THE IMPACT OF NEW LABOUR ON THE LIVES OF DISABLED PEOPLE

List any changes that may have occurred to benefit disabled people since the Labour Party came to power in 1997.

The present Labour Government under Tony Blair came into power in May 1997 and, as we write, is in its third term. New Labour is very different from the Old Labour of Beveridge's day and has largely left the health and social care reforms of the Conservative Party intact (Blakemore 1998). It has, however, sought to construct a Third Way between Old Labour and the New Right. New Labour stresses the need to reduce expenditure and increase choice and efficiency, but also emphasizes equal opportunities, social justice and social cohesion, it has, for instance, strengthened the Disability Discrimination Act. Like the New Right, it stresses individual and family responsibility but places more emphasis on collective issues within society (Blakemore 1998).

Although the purchaser–provider split remains intact, partnership rather than competition is now emphasized with terms such as 'seamless services' and 'joined-up thinking' being used to imply greater collaboration among service providers. Words such as 'partnership' and 'empowerment' now pepper policy documents and legislation (see Chs 8 and 9). Primary care groups, rather than individual GPs, now have the responsibility of negotiating with hospital trusts, and competition and contracts have been reduced by placing an emphasis on co-operative, long-term arrangements. New Labour has also introduced national standards and guidelines in an attempt to enhance quality of health and social care. Organizations such as the National Institute for Clinical Excellence and the Social Care Institute for Excellence have been set up in an attempt to improve standards. Many of these changes have the potential to improve services for disabled people, for instance the Disability Discrimination Act (1995) now covers education and notions of a 'seamless service', 'partnership' and 'empowerment' could make services for disabled people more responsive and efficient. Only time will tell whether or not such improvements will occur.

CONCLUSION

> ### *Activity* 3.6
>
> ### THE RELEVANCE OF HISTORY IN THERAPY PRACTICE TODAY
>
> Spend a little time thinking about (or preferably discussing with colleagues or disabled people) the ways in which this chapter may be useful in understanding therapy practice with disabled people now. What insights have you gained by reading about the history of developing practice?

In this chapter we have explored the history of the physiotherapy and occupational therapy professions in relation to their role with disabled people. It is clear that these and similar professions have developed in accordance with government policy and have been particularly influenced by the First and Second World Wars and the establishment of the welfare state. Recent social welfare policy has provided new challenges for physiotherapists and occupational therapists who work with disabled people, but the system of welfare is still very restrictive and the fundamental relationship of inequality between therapists and disabled people remains. It is impossible to appreciate fully the depth of prejudice against disabled people without a thorough understanding of their history, but it is only in recent times that this history has started to be told.

The history of physiotherapy and occupational therapy in relation to disabled people shows that, although these professions have undoubtedly helped in some instances, their presence in the lives of disabled people has been highly problematic because of the unequal professional/ client relationship and the 'social control' function that therapists and other professionals undertake. It is only in recent times that disabled people have had sufficient voice to influence social policy and practice. In doing so practices that were said to be caring are now labelled abusive, for example institutionalization and excessive medical treatment (French & Swain 2001). Disabled people have been assisted, to a limited extent, by such legislation as the Disability Discrimination Act (1995) and Human Rights Act (1998), which cover many aspects of health and social care, but their struggle for full control over their lives in all its aspects has only just begun.

Chapter **4**

Servicing the body

CHAPTER CONTENTS

In this chapter we will examine the role of biomedicine in the lives of disabled people. We will begin with a brief sojourn into the history of Western medicine where it will be seen that biomedicine (viewing health and illness solely in biological terms) only recently gained a dominant position. We will then move on to consider the pitfalls and benefits that biomedicine has brought to the lives of disabled people and the challenges that disabled people have directed at this approach. In relation to disability, the biomedicine approach is usually referred to as the medical model and is frequently contrasted with the social model of disability as we discussed in Chapter 2.

THE RISE OF THE BIOMEDICAL MODEL

Theories of health and illness before the 19th century were highly complex and contained many elements including religion, astronomy, anatomy and physiology. There was also a sound appreciation of how mood and environmental factors could influence health and wellbeing. Physical treatments (such as surgery and herbalism), advice (about diet and exercise) and sociopolitical action (such as quarantine during infectious disease) were practised. During epidemics and pandemics of plague, for example, people's movements were restricted, refuse was burned and the streets were cleaned. These measures appear very modern but at the same time healers openly prayed for their patients and behaviour such as gambling was strictly forbidden as the plague was thought to be a manifestation of the anger of god (de Renzi 2004).

Biomedicine started to emerge in the 18th century but at that stage it was far from monolithic. There were many rival schools of thought which were equally as powerful (Porter 1997, Saks 2005). Thus medicine was pluralistic with no notion of 'orthodox' and 'alternative' as we have today. Healers who could access a university education did, however, gradually gain power through the process of professionalization. This culminated in the passing of the Medical Registration Act in 1858 which secured their registration and dominance. The Act did not prevent other practitioners from working but they were marginalized as registration was necessary for employment in establishments run by the state, such as hospitals. This situation is similar today with many 'alternative' and 'complementary' practitioners seeking registration to work within the NHS (Heller 2005).

These changes can be viewed in the context of the Enlightenment (a period characterized by a belief in reason and the power of science) and the growth of capitalism. With the coming of the Industrial Revolution doctors worked in league with the state to monitor and control the population in the interests of the wealthy capitalist class; for example doctors had the power to place people considered to be disorderly or unproductive in asylums (Andrews 2005). Medicine was not very effective at this time, and could be hazardous, so the success of the physicians in reaching their privileged position over other healers was largely political.

The Medical Registration Act (1858) produced a medical elite. The necessity of having a university education precluded women (who comprised the majority of healers before the Act) and the bulk of the population who had neither the resources nor the education to attend university. It is only in recent years that women have entered medical school in similar numbers to men. The registered physicians launched many attacks on other healers, for instance through their journals, which further served to separate them and make them distinct. The professional association also developed an ethical code which prevented registered physicians from associating with other healers: indeed to do so could mean removal from the medical register. These measures led to further separation and elitism.

The situation for nurses was very different from that of doctors in the mid 19th century. As Rhodes (2004:164) explains:

> Nursing was carried out by women from a wide range of social backgrounds, from those caring for their own children, to inmates of the workhouse system nursing fellow paupers, to elite 'sisters' in charge of wards in large hospitals. While the latter group were distinguished by their experience, most nurses had little training.

Nursing did gradually emerge as a profession in its own right: state registration, for instance, was granted in 1919, but the gendered nature of nursing, with its close association with domestic work and caring, made professionalization very difficult and even today the nursing profession struggles to gain autonomy from medicine (Rhodes 2004).

By the mid 19th century the biomedical model had become dominant in Western medicine. The body was viewed as a complex machine and anatomy, physiology and the study of disease were given maximum importance. Far more attention was paid to the body than the mind, which were regarded as distinct entities, and an extensive education in the 'hard' sciences was deemed necessary. There was a focus on the disease rather than on the person, or the person's environment, and a quest to conquer or cure. Doctors also started making judgements about what should be regarded as 'normal' and 'pathological'. Modern inventions such as the stethoscope and microscope aided these pursuits, and various discoveries, for example of micro-organisms, gave the newly formed medical profession growing credibility, prestige and power.

In recent years it has been recognized that the biomedical model is very narrow in its scope. Porter (1997:7) states that:

> Whereas most traditional healing systems have sought to understand the relations of the sick person to the wider cosmos and to make readjustments between individual and world, or society and world, the western medical tradition explains sickness principally in terms of the body itself – its own cosmos.

The position of biomedicine has been challenged in the last 20 years by an upsurge in alternative and complementary practices (Cant 2005). Modern medicine has also started to consider the psychosocial needs of patients. General practitioners, for example, sometimes employ counsellors, though in this case it is interesting to note that the mind and the body are still treated separately, requiring the ministration of different professionals.

As biomedicine became dominant, patients and doctors no longer shared the same knowledge which led to an unequal power relationship between them. As Stewart et al (2003:192) state:

> The conventional medical model ... allows physicians to remain comfortably distant from patients and their problems. Also, if doctors do their best (biologically speaking), and their patients do not improve, the physician need feel no blame. If the patient did not 'comply' with the doctor's 'orders' then the lack of improvement can be blamed on the patient.

It should be realized, however, that until the introduction of the NHS in 1948, doctors charged fees which many people could not afford. This had the effect of maintaining 'home remedies' and the services of 'alternative healers' although the biomedical model gradually gained ground.

THE POWER AND SHORTCOMINGS OF THE BIOMEDICAL MODEL

 Activity 4.1

RECOVERY FROM ILLNESS

The biomedical model has claimed important successes in the history of medicine, and continues to do so. Until recent years it went largely unchallenged.

Think of two occasions when you have been helped by the biomedical approach. Was it enough, or was your recovery made possible or easier by other factors?

There are many examples you could have given of where the biomedical approach has been helpful. Perhaps you fractured a bone and had it fixed by a surgeon under anaesthetic, perhaps you were given antibiotics for an infection, or some analgesics for a migraine or toothache. Biomedicine is particularly successful in dealing with short-term, acute illnesses and injuries. It is, however, also important in the control of chronic diseases, for example insulin for people with diabetes, pain relief for people with arthritis and (more controversially; see Pilgrim & Rogers 1999) drug therapy for people in mental distress. Sometimes a fast and accurate diagnosis is vitally important in saving lives or reducing the impact of disease, for example the recognition that meningitis frequently begins with flu-like symptoms and a rash.

You may have considered, however, that despite the power of the bio-medicine approach you were also helped by the behaviour of the health professional, his or her communication skills and whether you were adequately consulted. In recent years the psychosocial aspects of health and illness have been recognized and have gradually gained a place in the curriculum of healthcare professionals including therapists (French & Sim 2004). Engel (1977) first proposed the biopsychosocial model which, as well as focusing on biological issues, acknowledges psychological and social factors. Sim & Smith (2004) discuss the biopsychosocial model in relation to pain and Reynolds (2004a) relates it to chronic illness. The World Health Organization's *International Classification of Impairments, Disabilities and Handicaps* (1980) also reflects a biopsychosocial approach. Thomas (2002:41) believes, however, that 'In the domain of rehabilitation services, the biomedical perspective on disability continues to have a weighty presence in training and practice'. It is also the case that the biopsychosocial model focuses on the individual and lacks a political dimension. In that respect it fails to connect with the social model of disability which we discussed in Chapter 2.

Going back to your experience of the biomedical approach, it may also be the case that non-medical people (family and friends, or cleaners and porters in the hospital) helped you as much, or more, in your recovery than the health professionals, through practical, psychological or social help and support.

Activity 4.2

BIOMEDICAL ADVANCES AND HEALTH

Think of at least two biomedical advances that you consider have helped many thousands of people. Are there any alternative ways of viewing these achievements?

You may have thought of the following developments, though many others could be added:

- Antibiotics.
- Anaesthetics.
- Radiotherapy and chemotherapy.
- Vaccination and inoculation.
- Joint replacement surgery.

- Open heart surgery.
- Insulin for people with diabetes.
- Analgesics.

All of these developments are important. In years gone by people endured surgery without anaesthetics and the skill of the surgeon was measured in terms of how fast he could perform the operation (Schlich 2005). People died or were impaired by infections which can now be cured by antibiotics. One of the most common causes of blindness until recent times, for example, was conjunctivitis and infections such as this still cause much impairment in many parts of the world (Stone 1999). People now live full and productive lives with diabetes, and epidemics such as poliomyelitis and diphtheria no longer occur in the Western world. Other viruses and bacteria which can cause death and impairment have, however, evolved, for example the HIV virus that leads to AIDS, so the problem of infectious disease has not be eradicated.

The glory bestowed on the medical profession for the control of infectious disease has, however, been questioned. The reason for this scepticism is that much of the decline in morbidity and mortality from infection occurred before any effective medical treatment was available and was due to improved diet and social conditions such as housing and sanitation. McKeown (1979) and Sagan (1987) give detailed evidence to illustrate this point. Mortality from tuberculosis, for example, declined sharply before the introduction of antibiotics and the BCG inoculation. A similar pattern can be seen for measles, whooping cough, poliomyelitis and diphtheria. Social reform does, therefore, have a greater impact on health than medicine though this is generally under-emphasized. Talking of psychiatry, Pilgrim & Rogers (1999:4) state that:

> The illness framework is the dominant framework in mental health services because psychiatry is the dominant profession within those services. However, its dominance should not be confused with its conceptual superiority.

Disabled people have benefited from medical advances which are underpinned by the biomedical model and many would, indeed, have died without them. Frontera (2006) stresses the reduction in mortality, due to medical intervention, from accidents and both acute and chronic diseases. Similarly, Oliver et al (1988) highlight the high mortality rate of people with spinal cord injuries before the advent of specialist units following the Second World War. Thus, it can be argued that medical advances have 'created' more disabled people and enabled them to live longer.

An alternative perspective on medicine is its tendency to cause ill-ness and impairment. This is termed 'iatrogenic medicine' (meaning 'physician produced'). Illich (1975) views iatrogenic medicine in phys-ical terms (for example addiction to barbiturates, surgical accidents, unnecessary treatment and infection contracted while in hospital) and in social and psychological terms (for example the dependency of people on medical professionals and their subsequent loss of coping skills). Coleman (1988:46) states:

> Survey after survey has shown that if you develop fresh symp-toms after being treated by your doctor then the chances are that your new symptoms will have been caused by the treatment given to you for your original problem.

The 'side effects' of the treatment may, however, be preferable to the symptoms of the disease or may prolong the person's life, for instance chemotherapy for cancer. The crucial point is that the person receiving the treatment should be fully informed and involved in whatever decisions are made. Coleman (1988) highlights the anxiety created by monitoring and preventative measures, such as mammograms and cervical smears, as well as the physical damage the tests may do and the tendency for people who are being monitored to become less vigilant. If people are told that they have a medical condition they may also change their behaviour and start to act like patients when this is unnecessary (Fitzpatrick 2001).

Environmental factors are very important in the creation of disease and impairment. It has repeatedly been shown that accidents, acute and chronic illness and mental distress are far more prevalent among people who are poor and who lack resources (Talley 2004). This is particularly stark in the majority (under-developed) world where 100 million people are impaired through malnutrition, including 250 000 children who go blind each year as a result of vitamin A deficiency (Stone 1999). Environmental factors (and perhaps medicine to a small extent) have also enabled more people to live into old age with a subse-quent rise in the number of people with impairments.

DISABILITY AND THE BIOMEDICAL MODEL

Despite the benefits of medical advances for some disabled people, they are often highly critical not only of the treatment they receive but of the way healthcare professionals communicate with them. Reynolds (2004a:19b) relates this to the dominance of the biomedical model:

> A substantial barrier to communication within the healthcare and therapy context is the traditional biomedical view of illness and

disability. This conceptual model presents the body in terms of a complex machine requiring attention when parts and processes function 'abnormally'. Whilst this viewpoint has undoubtedly led to a huge growth in biological knowledge and an awesome capacity to intervene medically in certain biological processes, it has distracted attention away from the importance of the communication processes occurring between professionals and clients. The biomedical conceptualisation of disease and impairment has traditionally encouraged clinicians to listen to clients only in so far as they can shed clues on their pathology and thereby contribute to an effective diagnosis.

It has been argued by French & Swain (2004) that listening is not enough and that communication between disabled people and health professionals requires an equalization of power within the relationship.

A central criticism of the biomedical model in relation to disability is that it is misplaced and misused. This will be explored in Activity 4.3.

 ### *Activity* 4.3

THE BIOMEDICAL MODEL AND 'NON–MEDICAL' IMPAIRMENTS

I (Sally) was born with a visual impairment caused by the absence of the macula on the retina of both eyes. The macula is a small group of cells (cones) which are responsible for fine visual acuity, central vision and colour vision. The visual impairment that results from an absence of the macula is severe and cannot be corrected. I am colour blind, can only read the top letter of the optician's chart (with as much correction as possible) and have no central vision. I am also photophobic and see very little in bright sunlight. Although I have very useful vision, I am registered blind and use visual aids such as a strong magnifying glass and a monocular (small telescope). I also use a white stick in certain situations such as crossing busy roads and I am eligible for a guide dog. The condition is non–progressive, with no medical treatment available, and yet ophthalmologists (eye specialists) have been prominent in my life, especially as a child.

What, if anything, do you consider the purpose of their involvement to be?

You may have thought that I would need to see an ophthalmologist in order for my visual impairment to be correctly diagnosed. In fact this particular impairment, though very rare in younger people, is visible with an ophthalmoscope and was readily diagnosed by the optician.

Other causes of visual impairment, such as albinism, may be similarly obvious although in other instances it may be necessary for an ophthalmologist to make the initial diagnosis.

In the early years of my childhood low vision aids had not been developed but I was helped a little with spectacles and I received the usual care from the optician. The only thing I remember about visits to the ophthalmologist was that the drops that were put in my eyes made my sight very much worse for several hours. Nothing was done during these consultations except looking in my eyes and attempting (in a rather desperate way) to get me to see more than I could.

A major role that the ophthalmologist played in my childhood was to decide that, at the age of nine, I should attend a residential boarding school for partially sighted girls. This was despite the fact that I was managing well in a small, country primary school with just thirty children. I suspect that the ophthalmologist knew little about child care, education or the social ramifications of removing a child from family and community. The school that I attended was an abusive institution with a very poor academic record (see French 1996b) which had implications in my later life.

Many disabled people have questioned the role of doctors and other healthcare professionals in non-medical areas of their lives such as education (French 2004). This issue is, however, broader than disability. In the 1970s, Freidson (1970) and Illich (1975) spoke about the 'medicalization of life'. This process, they proposed, de-skills and disempowers people and, by mystifying the causes of disease, enhances the power of medical 'experts' to intervene in non-medical domains. Zola (1972) views the medical profession as replacing other institutions such as the church, and Conrad & Schneider (1980) believe that the process of medicalization depoliticizes moral and social problems. Doyal (1998) speaks of the medicalization of childbirth, Katz (1998) of the medicalization of death and Scull (1979) of the medicalization of madness. Moynihan & Smith (2005) contend that it is easy to create new diseases and new treatments from normal aspects of life such as ageing, unhappiness and sexuality.

Talking of disability Barnes et al (1999b:195–6) state:

This 'medicalisation of disability' transformed the lives of disabled people. The medical interest was extended to include the selection of educational provision for disabled children, the assessment and allocation of work for disabled adults, the determination of the eligibility of welfare payments and the prescription of technical aids and equipment.

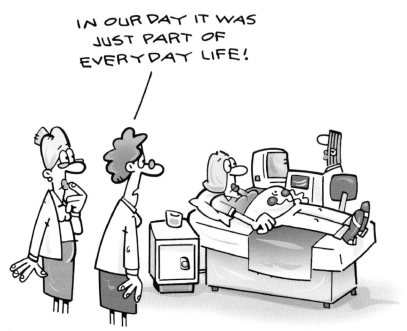

(From Porter S 2005 Dictionary of Physiotherapy, Oxford, Elsevier, 206)

At the school I attended we were regularly seen by an ophthalmologist but, as there was no medical intervention possible for my impairment (or for that of most of the other children) nothing of any consequence resulted. I do remember, however, repeatedly asking for my lenses to be tinted (as some of the other children's lenses were) to reduce my photophobia, but this was always denied and it was not until I had left school, and could take matters into my own hands, that the benefit of this was confirmed. There was no consultation or recognition of our own considerable knowledge and expertise. As Hughes (2002:58) states, 'The process of locating disability within the disciplinary scope of medicine has influenced profoundly the state of knowledge about it.'

Contact lenses and low visual aids were being developed at this time and we were used as 'experimental' subjects. This may have helped some people, and may have been a necessary stage in the development of this technology, but for many children the experience was distressing, as the following quotation shows:

> They expected you to cope and I didn't cope very well. I could wear them for a couple of hours but I was supposed to wear them for eight. I couldn't, my eyes wouldn't tolerate them although they did improve my sight. I had to sit there with them hurting and my eyes would be really blurry but there was no way I could

take them out, nobody seemed at all sympathetic, the attitude was that you were lucky to be chosen. They weren't like modern contact lenses, they covered the whole eye, they were really thick and heavy. I don't know who paid for the wretched things but if you had them you were supposed to wear them because they were expensive. I suppose we were a group of young people with different eye conditions who they could try them out on. When I left I gave them up straight away they were that uncomfortable.

(French 1996b:24–25)

This example shows that disabled children have been used experimentally for the benefit of medicine and related professions. Undoubtedly they would have profited themselves on some occasions, and many people benefit from contact lenses now, but nonetheless, disabled children had no choice about their participation in these developments even when it was clearly unpleasant. The pursuit of the biomedical approach is to cure or at least to approximate people to 'normality'. Contact lenses sometimes did improve people's sight and, as that was the goal, the fact that they were painful was considered irrelevant. Physically disabled children had similar experiences at the hands of health professionals, for example being operated upon repeatedly, spending years in hospital against their will and enduring painful treatments (see Ch. 3).

After leaving school, when I had more control of my life, I saw very little of ophthalmologists. However, like most disabled people, I have sometimes been forced to go through health professionals for non-medical concerns. I have, for instance, had to ask my GP for a letter to enable me to have extra time in an examination (despite my registration as blind) and, in a recent university post, I was compelled to go through the occupational nurse to sort out my computer needs – her knowledge of visual impairment and specialist computer equipment was slight! Although my eye condition is unlikely to change, I was put on a three month waiting list to see an ophthalmologist in order to obtain a replacement for a low vision aid which was old and damaged. This wait was impossible as I needed it for work so I bought my own – an option which would not be available to many disabled people. It struck me that the cost of the ophthalmologist's time would have amply covered the cost of the low vision aid. This is an example of 'gatekeeping' which disabled people find so frustrating. Finkelstein (2004:207), for example, relates the story of a bathroom rail he had fitted following a stroke:

She was absolutely adamant that no payment could be made because I had fitted the rail without going through the right procedures. Bewildered by this apathetic response to an initiative, that undoubtedly saved the 'caring' professions time and money, I asked if I should now have the rail removed so that social services could fit a new one according to correct procedures? Any independent spirit I might have audaciously expressed was swiftly crushed. With the confidence of a modernised professional I was told in no uncertain terms that if I did that I would go on a waiting list for the replacement.

Although my life has been adversely affected by medical professionals, even though my eye condition is not amenable to any medical treatment, this is nothing in comparison to some disabled people, particularly those with learning difficulties. Even in the absence of any known pathology, the problems people with learning difficulties experience have been explained predominantly in biological and medical terms. This was made explicit in 1948 when the NHS took over the administration of mental handicap institutions. Not only was the care inadequate, it was also dehumanizing and abusive (Ryan & Thomas 1990). A common punishment for women, for instance, was scrubbing floors. A woman interviewed by Potts & Fido (1991:60) recalled:

> They used to make you scrub from one end t'other. And if you didn't do it proper, you had to do it over. Sometimes if we didn't do it, we didn't get anything to eat. They once put me to bed without any tea.

Some people stayed in these institutions for many years, or indeed a lifetime, being made to work without pay, being forcibly segregated from people of the opposite sex and being denied all their rights as citizens (Potts & Fido 1991). Despite this, any problems they had were interpreted in terms of biology rather than the inadequacies of the institutions themselves. Oswin (2000:144), looking back at the time she spent working with disabled children in long-term hospitals, writes:

> Not only nurses, but doctors were disagreeable about any criticism of long-stay hospitals. They said that the children in Special Care Wards needed to live in hospitals because they 'required constant medical and nursing care'. My answer was to point out that the children never actually received any 'medical and nursing care' and that their general health was suffering because of neglect. It amazed me how nurses and doctors constantly denied that the children were neglected both physically and emotionally.

Walmsley (2006a) concludes that most people in mental handicap hospitals were there for social rather than medical reasons.

Activity 4.4

THE BIOMEDICAL MODEL AND 'MEDICAL' IMPAIRMENTS

I (John) was diagnosed as diabetic 12 years ago when I was in my late forties. I became increasingly ill over the summer months – loss of weight, loss of appetite, extreme thirst and a sore throat. Knowing nothing about diabetes I consulted my GP about the sore throat. He conducted blood and urine tests and I remember his words clearly: 'You've sugar coming out of your ears'. I was sent to the diabetes clinic where I was told that I had Type 1 diabetes, often referred to as 'younger diabetes'. Type 1 is usually inherited and diagnosed in childhood. Ninety to 95% of people with diabetes have Type 2. I have no family history of the condition and have never been offered a reason as to why I contracted what is classified as a 'chronic disease'. This, however, was the start of regular contact with medical professionals.

What do you consider the purposes and consequences of their involvement to be?

The initial purpose is quite obvious: diagnosis and control of the medical condition and, ultimately, survival. I have regular injections of insulin to control my blood sugar levels. Without medical intervention my health would undoubtedly have continued to deteriorate resulting in further impairments and ultimately death. Like many disabled people my survival has been dependent on medical intervention.

The direct consequence is most obviously the quantity of contact with the medical profession and with this the subtle, and not so subtle, reverberations for myself and my life. At the heart of this is control: control of my body, of course, but also control of my life. I can only give a few examples, but the scene was set at that first diagnostic meeting. The consultant reassured me that I would be able to lead a 'normal life'. He told me that many of his diabetic patients do the Great North Run. Running a marathon, or jogging of any kind, is not, however, part of my 'normal life' nor is it a normality I aspire to. In more formal terms, my GP has become a 'gatekeeper'. The most obvious example is that I now have to renew my driving licence every three years and I need a medical certificate to do so.

I have been regularly subjected to 'blanket' policy and practice. One was the policy of all people with diabetes being prescribed statin drugs to lower cholesterol levels. It is a long story but basically I had an extremely adverse response, experiencing the side effects that I now know others have experienced, including loss of appetite, tiredness and tinnitus. A year of my life was dominated by coping with these so-called 'side effects' and slowly coming to realize that the drug was causing the problems. This is a clear example of iatrogenic medicine which was discussed above. Though I did consult doctors about this, at no point was I told about the possibility of side effects. I eventually took myself off the drug. When I told the doctor at my next appointment he looked through my records and said that my cholesterol levels were not that bad anyway and that I need not be taking the drug. Thus I was prescribed statins on the basis of policy, not assessment of my individual needs. Overall, my relationship with the medical profession is a dilemma. On the one hand I require medical intervention. On the other, I do not want my life to be determined and controlled by medical professionals and their presumptions about me.

The biomedical model has underpinned a great deal of research on disabled people with the current emphasis being on genetics (Kerr & Shakespeare 2002). We will discuss the topic of research in greater detail in Chapter 11, but it is important to realize at this point that research underpinned by the biomedical model has been *on* rather than *with* disabled people and has done nothing to address the oppression they experience or to investigate the disabling environment. Research which involves disabled people and which has an 'outward' orientation has, however, been promoted and practised by disabled researchers and their allies and, over the past 15 years, a body of literature on disability research has grown (see Barnes & Mercer 1997, Walmsley & Johnson 2003). Much of this research has been written into books and publications where disabled people have spoken for themselves (see Atkinson et al 1997, French et al 2006, Parr et al 1997).

Some health professionals have moved away from the biomedical model and base their practice on the biopsychosocial model, thereby attempting to adopt a holistic approach. Ewles & Simmett (2003) believe that a holistic approach to health care has the following dimensions: physical, mental, social, emotional, spiritual and societal. It is important, however, that both the interaction and intervention are on disabled people's terms and from their perspective, or the medicalization of their lives is likely to result. Finlay (2000a) relates the concept of holism to team work, where each member of the team brings something different and of value to the client. She admits, however, that this is not always achieved and can lead to fragmentation as the following quotation from a disabled woman shows (French 2004:101):

Another problem is lack of liaison between occupational therapists in the community and in the hospital. I had multiple problems, they don't talk to each other. One would promise me one thing, the next would say that I couldn't have it and another would modify it. It's very, very confusing because you really don't know what's going to happen.

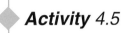

Activity 4.5

MODELS OF HEALTHCARE AND THERAPY PRACTICE

Think about your education and practice as a physiotherapist or an occupational therapist. When working with disabled people how far is your education and practice underpinned by the biomedical model? If you consider your work to be holistic, how far do you involve the patients and clients in the decisions that are made and how do you safeguard against the problems disabled people face in their contact with health professionals which were highlighted in Activities 4.3 and 4.4?

CONCLUSION

The lives of disabled people have largely been defined in medical and biological terms. This has been partly responsible for the dehumanization and abuse of disabled people and the restrictive lives they have endured. It can be argued very strongly that therapists need knowledge of biological and medical factors in order to work effectively and safely in their roles, but these factors should never be allowed to dominate the lives that disabled people wish to lead. Therapists need to work in collaboration with disabled people on an equal basis and should be prepared to learn about disability in all its complexity, both formally and from the disabled people they meet. Simply applying a biopsychosocial model, or attempting to work holistically, is not enough and can do great harm if professional power comes to dominate wider aspects of disabled people's lives.

Chapter **5**

Disabled people's experiences of health care

In this chapter we will be concentrating on the experiences of disabled people who have been the recipients of healthcare services. This has not been a central concern of healthcare professionals and information such as this is not reported or discussed in standard therapy textbooks. We have, therefore, turned to the disability studies literature to find out what disabled people have to say about their experiences of health care and their encounters with healthcare professionals. This information will be drawn from the present day and the recent past. Using the voice of disabled people to inform the discussion, we will also consider how healthcare services and the relationship between healthcare professionals and disabled people can be improved.

DISABLED PEOPLE'S EXPERIENCES OF HEALTH CARE

Those at the receiving end of professional services sometimes find themselves in opposition to professionals. Such people include women who may feel that doctors are taking control of their bodies, in childbirth for example (Doyal 1998), and people from ethnic minority groups who may perceive professionals as ethnocentric, racist and lacking in cultural awareness and sensitivity (Ahmad & Atkin 1998).

Disabled people have both good and bad experiences of health care and healthcare professionals. Reading about their positive experiences is not, of course, difficult but reading about their negative experiences may cause uncomfortable feelings and a tendency to ignore or reject what is said. It is important to remember that while healthcare professionals are not powerless to bring about changes to the way disabled people are treated, they are, nonetheless, enmeshed in a broad system of oppressive practices and discrimination against disabled people – based, for example, on monetary constraints and historical factors such as institutionalization – of which they have limited responsibility or control as individuals. Reynolds (2004b:17b) believes that:

> While many individual therapists value empowering relationships, they encounter significant barriers because of the ways in which health, disability, normality and well-being are defined in the health care system, and in Western culture more generally.

Disability studies (the social, political and cultural analysis of disability) is also virtually absent from the educational curriculum of healthcare professionals who, therefore, have little opportunity to learn about the meaning of disability within a formal educational setting (Whalley Hammell 2006).

We recognize that the readers of this book will be motivated to assist disabled people and to serve as a positive force to improve their lives. To achieve this we believe that an essential first step is to listen to what disabled people say about their experiences of health care, both good and bad. Unless professionals adapt to the needs and wishes of disabled people and become more involved in their struggle for citizenship, it can be argued that their role is very limited. As Williams (1996:200) states:

> … if the problem is not the need of the individual to adapt to the impairment, but rather the complex process of negotiating the interactions of which daily life is created, then the role of professional experts as people who do things to the impaired body is clearly limited.

REFLECTING ON PROBLEMS

Activity 5.1

PROBLEMS WITH HEALTH CARE – DISABLED PEOPLE'S EXPERIENCES

Read the following quotations from disabled people who are talking about their experiences of health care. Make a few notes on what you consider to be the two major themes that emerge from these quotations.

How many hours did I spend in those endless corridors learning to 'walk'
before returning home and promptly settling into a more active and
rewarding life in a wheelchair?

(Finkelstein 1990:6)

After being diagnosed as deaf, I tried to get on with my childhood while being
constantly interrupted to sit in a hospital chair straining for the slightest
possible noise ... which had no meaning and was not of the slightest interest.

(Heaton 1998:12)

I remember speech therapy being a lot of hard work and I can remember
getting extremely fed up. I got to a situation where I hated eating because at
every mealtime the speech therapist would come into the dining room to
supervise us saying, 'Remember what we talked about, remember about your
swallowing, remember how to drink' ... OK it's good to do it while you're
actually eating something, rather than talking about it in theory, but when
you're doing it at every mealtime, and your parents have been told so they do
it at home, you get to a point when you think, 'Wouldn't it be nice to just sit
and enjoy your food!?' You get to a point where you've eaten a meal and you
can't remember what you've eaten – it becomes a technical exercise ... I do
question the years of not enjoying food and getting to a point when I dreaded
mealtimes. But now I think, 'This is me, this is what I do, I've made a mess on
my shirt and I don't give a toss, it can be cleaned up, just eat for the pleasure
of eating and to hell with the rest.' ... You reach a point when you say 'tough!'
If I spill my coffee I'm now more interested in the pretty pattern it makes.

(French 2004:104)

The arm was better when it was done but as time's gone on it's just gone
back to how it was ... what did annoy me to be honest was they never said
this could happen, at the beginning it was, oh it will be wonderful. Looking
back if I knew then what I know now I would not have had the operation
done. It messed up so many things at the time.

(Middleton 1999:21)

I couldn't see the point of all those agonising exercises. I was never very
good at accepting the fact that things I didn't like could be 'good for me'
and the physiotherapist managed to do a really good job of making me a
conscientious objector for the rest of my life.

(Begum 1994:48)

I hated learning speech – hated it – I felt so stupid having to repeat the
s,s,s ... Every time I got it wrong. I had to do it all over again and I was
asking myself, 'Why do I have to keep going over and over it? I don't
understand what it all means!' ... It was just so stupid, a waste of time when
I could have been learning more important things.

(Corker 1996:92)

Their responses towards me varied greatly, some showed great compassion,
while others showed complete indifference. I had no way of communicating
the fact that I was a bright, intelligent, whole human being. That is what
hurt the most.

(Boazman 1999:18–19)

Contained within these quotations are two very strong and persistent themes. The first is that disabled people do not necessarily believe that medical treatment and what it might achieve is the most important thing within their lives. A second theme relates to the lack of power disabled people have over their lives, especially during childhood. As Oliver (1990:92) states:

> Medical need still predominates over educational: disabled children still have operations (necessary and unnecessary) that fit in with the schedule of surgeons and hospitals rather than educational programmes. Children are still taken out of classes for doctor's appointments or physiotherapy and the school nurse is still a more influential figure than the teachers.

Despite the distress and disruption medical treatment may cause, disabled people are under considerable pressure to go through with it. If they do assert themselves they frequently meet with resistance or even hostility, as the following quotations illustrate:

> I've known a few people who, as adults, have refused to walk even though they could because it's just not worth the effort. And people have got angry with them, often. They've been labelled lazy and all sorts of things. They're definitely considered odd if they choose to be in a wheelchair, in the same way that you're considered odd if you don't struggle to do something that you can actually do even though it takes you six hours.
>
> (Sutherland 1981:69)

> I came to realise that expending energy on having fun and living life are rather more important than preserving all one's energy and motivation for doing therapy and chasing dreams of cure.
>
> (Pound 2004:39)

> About two years ago I realised that my walking ability had deteriorated … so I talked to my GP who referred me to the physiotherapy department at my local hospital. She said, 'We can stop the deterioration provided you're willing to spend an hour a day working at it' and she didn't like it because I said I didn't feel that the work was worth it. I told her that I've got limited energy, some of my functions are not automatic, like when I'm talking I'm also trying to remember to swallow my saliva. When I'm walking I'm thinking 'left foot, right foot, left foot, right foot'. All those things are tiring. I said to her that I'm more interested in doing things that engage my mind and imagination, I'm not going to waste my energy going 'up down, up down'. She didn't like it and she wrote

me off as somebody she couldn't help rather than treating me as somebody she had helped by giving me some advice.

(French 2004:103)

It should be noted that in the third quotation the disabled person was not dissatisfied with the consultation with the physiotherapist, which he found useful, but he was disappointed in the physiotherapist's response when he declined to take her advice.

Not only can important areas of life be disrupted by medical intervention but the treatment itself can be very unpleasant. Furthermore the results of the treatment are sometimes short lived or less than satisfactory. Oliver, talking of the Peto system of treating children with cerebral palsy, goes as far as to liken it to abuse. He states (Oliver 1996:107):

If able-bodied children were taken from their local schools, sent to a foreign country, forced to take physical exercise for all their waking hours to the neglect of their academic, educational and social development, we would regard it as unacceptable and the children concerned would rapidly come to the attention of the child protection mafia. But in the lives of disabled children (and adults too) anything goes as long as you call it therapeutic.

Middleton (1999:41) makes a similar point:

What seems to have developed is an attitude towards the use of unproven treatment for disabled children which maintains that it may as well be tried, it can't do any harm since they are already impaired. This ignores the very real pain, discomfort and indignity that children suffer as a result of these experiences ... which non-disabled children would not be expected to.

Middleton is also critical of the way in which parents get caught up in financing and promoting unproven treatment because of a need to 'do all they can' for their disabled child.

The treatment that disabled people have sometimes received at the hands of professionals cannot be dismissed as benign or misguided. Serious physical, psychological and sexual abuses have all occurred (Westcott & Cross 1996). Mabel, a woman with learning difficulties, talks of the psychological abuse she experienced in a mental handicap hospital where she lived for many years (Brigham et al 2000:22):

I never said anything in the hospital because there was no point. Nobody listened, so why speak? If you spoke they told you to shut up, so I stopped saying anything. I didn't talk, it was a protest really rather than anything else. I only said two words 'yes' and 'no', and mostly I said 'no'!

REFLECTING ON SATISFACTION

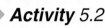 *Activity* 5.2

SATISFACTION WITH HEALTH CARE – DISABLED PEOPLE'S EXPERIENCES

The following quotations are from disabled people who have had positive experiences of therapy (French 2004). They are expressing satisfaction with the way therapists treated them as individuals, particularly in giving them control and considering their lives beyond the confines of biomedicine. After reading the quotations, reflect on your own practice as a therapist or therapy student and consider how far it would be possible to incorporate these positive aspects of therapy into your own role.

She said, 'Come in when you like and use all the equipment'. I was particularly lucky with my physio because she had the foresight to realise that that was what I needed for my recovery – to be in control ... She treated me like a person, she spoke to me like a person and not a patient. I felt in control and that gave me more confidence in myself.

(p. 96)

When I gave up work, and I was very, very involved in my work, my GP referred me to occupational therapy to try and get me to come to terms with it. They were very helpful. We set up a plan together. I was filling my time with hobbies and I was driven to finish every single task all the time just as if I was at work. We explored that together. They were very supportive and very helpful. They seemed to understand what I was feeling and we made very small goals. I kept a diary that we explored and worked from. It was very positive and made a big difference.

(p. 96)

I was in the physiotherapy department, they all knew me well, I was part of the furniture, and I remember saying to one of the physios, 'Why isn't there any counselling?' I said, 'There really should be counselling offered to people who've had strokes and who have communication problems.' I was doing a lot of moaning at that time because I was miserable and this physio said, 'Harry, I'm fed up with you moaning about this, I agree with you entirely but why don't you do something about it? Why don't you do a counselling course because I think you'd be really good at it?' She said, 'there's a real need for it and you have the personal qualities and experience to do it so stop moaning and do something about it'. I wandered around for weeks afterwards thinking 'I wonder' and 'maybe'. The thing that helped me so much was her belief that I could do it.

(p. 97)

In the first quotation the physiotherapist met the needs of the disabled person by giving her control – which would have meant relinquishing some of her own power and control. The physiotherapist realized that being in control, for this particular patient at least, was crucial for her recovery. The disabled person also noted that she was 'treated like a person and not a patient' which means that the physiotherapist managed to convey her interest in the disabled person as a complex individual with a past and a future rather than merely somebody with an impairment who needed treatment.

In the second quotation the occupational therapist supported the disabled person in rebuilding her life by helping her to come to terms with change and by focusing on the disabled person's own particular hobbies and desired lifestyle. There appears to have been maximum collaboration between them which gave power and control to the disabled person and involved the occupational therapist in relinquishing her own power and control while, at the same time, maximizing her ability to help.

The third quotation is more controversial as the physiotherapist speaks quite harshly to Harry, the disabled person. This may have been a risky strategy as it could have caused offence. However, Harry was well known to the physiotherapist and 'part of the furniture' in the physiotherapy department and it would seem that their relationship was sufficiently strong to accommodate this rebuke. What the physiotherapist said also contained a very positive message, that Harry was a capable adult with many valuable skills, experiences and attributes, not just a disabled person who needed treatment. The interaction with the physiotherapist had a profound effect upon Harry who went on to become a fully qualified counsellor specializing in people with aphasia.

It is very often the case that the experiences disabled people have in their encounters with healthcare professionals are neither wholly good nor bad but a complex mix. This can be illustrated by the following examples given by three disabled women when they were pregnant. Alison Lapper, for instance, found that her GP was very supportive but that the Social Services staff were not. She explains (Lapper 2005:196, 198):

> I went to my GP … and she confirmed that I was pregnant. I told her about my situation and that I couldn't count on Tim or my family. She listened sympathetically and told me not to worry. If I wanted to have the baby she would support me 100 per cent. It was wonderful to hear a medical professional being so positive about my prospects. It helped my morale enormously … Alison (the GP) arranged a case conference with other professionals, such as occupational therapists, and social services to see whether they would be able to support me in any way, either during or after the pregnancy. Social services were particularly hard on me at that meeting. They said that I'd created the situation and would have to deal with it on my own. There was no money to help me.

The ideology of the eugenics movement, which we discussed in Chapter 3, underpins the message from Social Services to Alison Lapper, that, as a disabled woman, she really has no right to have a child.

Kate, a woman with mental health problems, encountered similar attitudes from a consultant psychiatrist when she was pregnant (The Open University 2002):

> One of the things that really added to our anxiety about our ability to cope was the attitude of a consultant psychiatrist. I was seeing him for the first time, as we'd moved to a different area, and I was asking advice on taking medication during pregnancy … his response to that was that we shouldn't have children, we'd be passing on defective genes, and he also said that if I became ill the child would be taken away 'no doubt about it' … It made me feel quite angry actually but also very anxious.

Mary, a physically disabled woman, experienced nothing but positive attitudes when she was pregnant with twins but her quotation shows that, without a full understanding of disability, this was not enough.

> I don't remember a single negative reaction to my being pregnant neither from family or friends, nor from the professionals … In retrospect their vision of being positive towards a disabled person was very much to treat me like any other mother … so actually they weren't addressing needs with me that it would have been wise to address particularly in relation to when I was actually delivering and also when I would be on the maternity unit. The fact that these things hadn't been addressed caused an awful lot of trouble really.
>
> (The Open University 2002)

REFLECTING ON ASSUMPTIONS

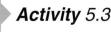

Activity 5.3

UNDERLYING ASSUMPTIONS IN THERAPY PRACTICE

Read the following quotations from disabled people and make some notes on the underlying assumptions that appear to underpin therapy practice and which may conflict with the perspectives of disabled people. How far does this apply to your own work as a therapist or therapy student?

What concerns me most of all is this focus on trying to make me 'normal'. I get that from all the therapists. I get a lot of referrals of 'this may help' and 'that may help'. They had a massive case conference before the adaptations – it was a case of 'how normal can we make her first? Are the adaptations necessary?' They deliberately didn't widen the bathroom door upstairs to try and make me walk to the toilet. I very deliberately leave the feet off my wheelchair to keep my legs moving – it's definitely helped to maintain the muscle tone – but they don't like this. I can't feel them so I have to be very careful as I've been known to run over my own feet. They don't like it for safety reasons, but you make choices – I go sailing and that could be dangerous ... Nobody thinks about the real world, it's all very purist.

(French 2004:103–104)

The staff were very keen that we all became proficient in the use of our artificial limbs. The add-on limbs were considered a fundamental aspect of our being able to function properly ... So when we were eating they always stood behind the tables and watched us to make sure we used them. They had great faith in those artificial limbs and thought that if we would only practice and use them regularly we would soon be picking up even the most delicate items without breaking or damaging them. But we all instinctively knew those sorry bits of metal were never going to fulfil their hoped-for potential.

(Lapper 2005:35)

There's a tremendous emphasis on a child who's had polio or whatever to walk, to be as able-bodied as possible. It's like standing up is infinitely better than sitting down, even if you're standing up in a total frame – metal straps and God knows what – that weighs a ton, that you can't move in, which hurts, takes hours to get on and off and looks ugly. It's assumed that that's what you want and that's what is best for you.

(Sutherland 1981:72)

What I did find incredibly difficult to come to terms with was somebody coming into my home and saying 'This needs to be done and this is how it's gong to be done.' I had no say whatsoever to the point where ... well one of the things is the front door which is completely flat because I'm in a wheelchair. I could cope with a small rise very easily and I demonstrated that I could manage. What happens now is that whenever you open the door the leaves blow in because it's so flat. I had quite a long argument, added to which the builder had difficulty finding such a flat front door.

(French 2004:100)

The ideologies of the health and caring professions have had a considerable impact on the lives of many disabled people, not only in terms of policy, practice and provision, but on the way disabled people have been defined (Swain et al 2004a). Professionals have viewed disabled people as tragic, deficient and inferior and have sought to eliminate them (through abortion and genetic engineering), remove them from society (through institutionalization) and to cure or approximate them to 'normal' (through surgery, drugs and rehabilitation). Professionals have the power to assess disabled people, to label them, to define their needs, to specify solutions and to evaluate outcomes. They also have the power to make moral judgements about disabled people and to control resources. This, together with a disabling physical and social environment, has served to keep disabled people in a dependent position within society (Oliver 1993).

The underlying assumption that struck us as the most persistent and powerful in these quotations was that disabled people should strive to be 'normal' and function as near like non-disabled people as possible. In many cases this appears to be the main goal of therapy which disabled people tend to reject as a goal. As Middleton (1999:42) remarks, 'Mobility is important, but it does not necessarily need to be achieved through walking, any more than communication has to be through the spoken word.' Finkelstein (2004) highlighted this issue when he protested against the slogan of the 1999 Occupational Therapy Day, *Able to Make you Able*. He contends that it is society, not disabled people, which needs to change and that 'making disabled people able' is a medical goal that is neither achievable nor desirable and is offensive to many disabled people. This leads us back to our earlier discussion of the social versus the medical model of disability in Chapter 2. Many disabled people have questioned the time, effort and expense involved in trying to make them 'normal' rather than changing the physical and social environment. Finkelstein (1990:6), for instance, asks:

> ... do you not think that we might better spend scarce resources making the world fit for disabled people rather than spending so much more trying to fit us into the able-bodied world?

The pressure to strive for 'normality' is one aspect of what has been referred to as the 'disabled role' (French 1994a, Sutherland 1981). The expectations of this role are that disabled people should struggle to be independent (in the narrow sense of looking after their own basic needs), should strive to emulate 'normality' and should passively accept and adjust to the situation they find themselves in without protest or complaint. Rejecting this role is likely to cause considerable conflict between disabled people and healthcare professionals. Oliver (1996:104) explains this using walking as an example:

> Non-walking, or rejecting nearly walking as a personal choice ... threatens the power of professionals. It exposes the ideology of normality and it challenges the whole rehabilitation enterprise.

It is clear from the quotations from disabled people in Activity 5.3 that the pressure to be 'normal' and 'independent' is placed on them as children and as adults. Talking of disabled children, Middleton (1999:40) states that:

Underpinning all this is the obsession of society with what constitutes normality. These treatments are not aimed at making the child happy, sociable, well or even comfortable but moulding them towards *physical acceptability*.

Holliday Wiley, who has Asperger's syndrome, reflects on the loss of self through attempting to be 'normal' (1999:95):

I meet who I am with a certain amount of sadness, for I often wonder what parts of me I had to leave behind before I came to this place in my life. Would I have been a better writer if I had allowed my skewed take on the world to find its way to paper ... If I had not been taught and encouraged to be as social as I now am, would I have found a different and more satisfying kind of individualised lifestyle? Would I have avoided my irritable bowel syndrome and panic attacks if I had not tried so hard to be normal?

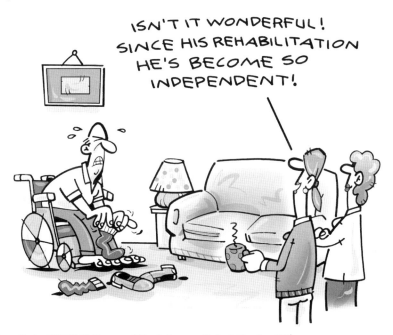

(From Porter S 2005 Dictionary of Physiotherapy, Oxford, Elsevier, 165)

Disabled children are particularly vulnerable as they lack control over their lives and their parents often collude with health professionals in their pursuit of 'normality' and 'independence'. Adults are thought to be the 'experts' and it is assumed that children do not understand the problems they face or have any solutions to offer (Davis 2004). It is clear from interviews with disabled children, however, that this is far from the truth (see Ballard & McDonald 1999, French & Swain 2004, French et al 2006).

The emphasis placed on 'normality' and 'independence' can have wide and adverse repercussions in the lives of disabled people. Because medical treatment is considered so important in the achievement of these goals it has a tendency to disrupt other substantial areas of life such as education and leisure. It can also cause feelings of embarrassment, inferiority and lack of self-esteem for disabled people. If the ability to walk, talk or eat in the conventional way is emphasized and given prominence, other ways of achieving communication, mobility and eating are devalued and even despised.

Morris (1993b) believes that the assumption that disabled people want to be 'normal', rather than just as they are, is one of the most oppressive experiences to which they are subjected. She rejects the view that it is progressive and liberating to ignore difference, believing that disabled people have a right to be both equal and different. She states, 'I do not want to have to try to emulate what a non-disabled woman looks like in order to assert positive things about myself. I want to be able to celebrate my difference not hide from it.' (Morris 1991:184). Similarly, as Pound (2004:43) states:

> The imposition of the importance of cure, and the implication that a person cannot be whole or good enough without a cure is in direct conflict with the self respect of people with disabilities.

In the first quotation in Activity 5.3 the issue of safety and the ability to take risks is raised. As health and safety legislation has tightened over the years disabled people have found themselves more and more restricted and, paradoxically, prevented from undertaking 'normal' tasks.

This quotation emphasizes the lack of control some disabled people have over their lives and highlights the underlying assumption that they are incompetent when it comes to making judgements about what is best for them. Similarly, the final quotation in Activity 5.3 shows that the disabled person is thought to lack competence regarding the design of her house and what she can and cannot do, or wishes to do, in the context of her life as a whole. Professionals have more power than disabled people to define disability and, as McKnight (1995) contends, there is no greater power than the right to define the problem. As noted in Chapter 4, the status of healthcare professionals also gives them the power to intervene in non-medical areas of disabled people's lives. The advice of a doctor or a therapist may, for example, be sought when decisions are made about the education or employment of disabled people with little or no consultation with disabled people themselves. In this way the lives of disabled people can become increasingly 'medicalized' even though the professionals have little knowledge or understanding of the issues involved.

Another problem that disabled people face in their encounters with healthcare professionals is communication. This can operate at different levels, as the following quotations show:

> Often I've found it difficult to follow specialists. They tend to shout, they know very little about communication with deaf people.
>
> (Sutherland 1981:125)

> When I came back for the negatives, oh it was terrible. He lifted them up to the light and he said to the nurse 'Macula degeneration in both eyes, sign a BDS form' or whatever it is. And then he turned to me and he said 'There's nothing we can do about it'. He said 'You'll always be able to see sideways but you've got no central vision.' … So I came home feeling very upset about it.
>
> (French et al 1997:37)

In the first example the problem is to do with lack of knowledge of a different method of communication and lack of appropriate help such as the services of a sign language interpreter. Similar problems have been experienced by visually impaired people (French et al 1997) and people with learning difficulties (O'Hara & Sperlinger 1997) who lack access to health information because their needs regarding communication are ignored. Healthcare services have been slow to make their premises, and the information they provide, accessible to disabled people despite the passing of the Disability Discrimination Act in 1995 (Clark 2002).

In the second quotation the problem is more to do with insensitivity and lack of empathy. In saying 'there's nothing we can do about it' the health professional is also demonstrating a very narrow, biomedical perspective and a lack of understanding of the meaning of disability. Although it is true that the loss of central vision in macular degeneration cannot be restored, there are many ways in which visually impaired people can be assisted to lead full and active lives and to enhance the sight they have. Disabled people frequently remark that medical professionals do not understand the implications of impairment. A person with albinism, interviewed by Roy & Spinks (2005:105) states that:

> … often you find that people who are experts in ophthalmology and perhaps experts in certain conditions, they will know the genetics and the physiology of a certain condition and prognosis and so on. But when it comes to the practical feelings and the

practical effects that people experience, they quite often are not so tuned in.

None of this is to say that disabled people do not want the help and expertise of healthcare professionals. Campbell & Oliver (1996:146) state:

> There are many disabled people who want really brilliant medical services because they need them for their lives. They need them in terms of pain control, they need them in terms of pressure sore treatment.

Pound (2004:46) values the technical expertise of therapists but found it insufficient to her rehabilitation:

> I still greatly value the technical knowledge and expertise that my physiotherapist shared with me … but in retrospect I also realise that this form of expertise alone did not move me forward. I valued the careful listening of therapists and non-therapists, and the challenge to view things differently that came from people who lived with disabilities themselves. Ultimately it was these people with their entirely different knowledge and understanding of the world of the 'other' that helped me to realise that my greatest steps in rehabilitation happened outside the therapy room.

Barnes & Mercer (2006:37) believe that impairment is significant in people's lives but that the ideology and practice of healthcare professionals demonstrates a lack of interest in disability and an 'extraordinary silence' about the existence and impact of disabling barriers.

CRITICAL REFLECTIONS ON CHANGING PRACTICE

Now that we have examined the commendations and criticisms disabled people have of healthcare professionals and some of the reasons why difficulties occur, it is time to consider how the situation can be improved. In the next activity we will turn again to disabled people's own experiences to discover more about what they value in therapeutic relationships and what advice they have to give to improve therapy services.

◆ *Activity 5.4*

IMPROVING THERAPY SERVICES – DISABLED PEOPLE'S PERSPECTIVES

From your experience of working with clients as a therapist or therapy student, what attributes do you think clients value in you as a therapist? Compare your ideas with those of a colleague.

Now read the following quotations from disabled people who have received therapy. These quotations are taken from eight interviews which focused on disabled people's experiences of physiotherapy, occupational therapy and speech and language therapy (French 2004). Make a list of everything the disabled people value about therapy and the skills and attributes they would hope to find in a therapist. You may also like to look back to Activity 5.2 where you considered similar issues.

The speech therapist was a very special type of person and she gave me a sense that I was being valued as a person. She listened and she gave me the answers that I was looking for. She built up my confidence somehow. What she did was tell me why she was doing therapy and what it was meant to achieve and she explained the purpose of what she was doing. Instead of the normal speech therapy scenarios that you would expect, she would try to connect it to my previous work as a manager so that I could relate to it. I felt she understood where I was coming from. That way I felt more in control and that gave me confidence in her as a therapist and in myself – it built up my self-confidence.

(p. 95–96)

It was one particular physiotherapist who came in the middle of the night and she was so helpful and made such a difference. She said, 'Try dropping your shoulders a little bit' and 'If you put a pillow in the back of your neck that will help.' I use the techniques all the time now, it seems a very small thing but it made a huge difference. On the whole physiotherapists back away because they think they can't do anything, whereas she approached it in a very different way. She realised that she didn't have to have 'hands on' at all, that is was something I could do for myself. It made an enormous difference. They are usually very physical and you are supposed to be very physical. It was a small suggestion together with emotional support.

(p. 97)

I liked my speech therapist, she was trying to improve my communication and I remember thinking, 'what a fantastic woman, what a fantastic job' ... She showed kindness, kindness is something that is not acknowledged enough. She was gentle and empathetic, I felt as if she was joining in with my struggle.

(p. 97)

I want them to say 'What sorts of things would help you to lead a full life in the context of your impairment? It's either 'you're disabled and what can we do to make you better?' or 'you're OK'. Nobody says 'What would make a better life?' That's what I would like.

(p. 104)

The biggest thing is about asking and not telling. They need to get into the habit of asking what would be helpful ... we respect them far more if we can have an equal partnership in the challenge we're both facing. I would expect a person to be trained to the task and have an excellent knowledge base, and I would expect to have an exchange of knowledge – theirs would be knowledge from their training and mine would be about my own body, and my life style. I would expect the therapist to hear me. I would expect them to be creative.

(p. 104)

How far did your ideas tally with those of the disabled people?

In some ways the message from disabled people to therapists is very simple. Disabled people want a warm, honest, empathetic and trusting relationship where they are treated as equal partners. The advice given in these quotations is similar to that of Belle Brown et al (2003:5–6) who advocate practice which is patient centred. They state:

> Patient-centred care presupposes several changes in the mindset of the clinician. First, the hierarchical notion of the professional being in charge and the patient being passive does not hold here. To be patient-centred the clinician must be able to empower patients, share the power in the relationship, and this means renouncing control which traditionally has been in the hands of the profession. This is the moral imperative in patient-centred practice.

Whalley Hammell (2006:197) states that 'What clients want is help to manage their impairments or illnesses so they can get on with what really matters: their roles, relationships and valued routines and occupations'. She goes on to challenge the claim that therapists are, at present, client centred:

> If the rehabilitation professions' everyday practices, research practices, theories, education programmes, modes of service delivery and professionalising strategies do not place clients' expressed needs at their centre, then they are not client-centred professions despite assertions to the contrary.
>
> (Whalley Hammell 2006:150)

It is important for therapists to realize that the goals and aspirations of disabled people vary enormously and may be very different from those typically set by professionals.

Although disabled people value the skill and expertise of therapists, they want their own expertise to be recognized and to work in collaboration with therapists. Brown (2000) states that clients have challenged the appropriateness of professional knowledge by insisting that their own knowledge of illness, impairment and disability is equally as valid as that of professionals. As Pound (2004:39), a disabled speech and language therapist, states:

> For me, another key milestone in acknowledging my strength and experience as a disabled person was the recognition that through my experience I had acquired an expertise that my doctors and therapists lacked and that I really could make a contribution. However for many years the uncertainty with which I experienced each day was no match for the clarity and certainty of medicine

and consequently I afforded my growing expertise little value or status.

Disabled people expect therapists to value them, listen to them, consult them and give them detailed information. They also value encouragement, emotional support and control over their own lives. Therapists who are gentle and kind, assertive on behalf of disabled people at vulnerable times, and who can link treatment to the disabled person's lifestyle and quality of life and can 'be themselves' are highly regarded. Pound (2004:46), talking of speech and language therapists, emphasizes the importance of the non-technical aspects of the client–therapist relationship. She states:

> Listening to clients discussing their likes and dislikes of individual therapy, it is often difficult to find features which relate to more technical aspects of language exercises. Most often they highlight time, space and a listening relationship as the features of therapy which they most value. It is this intense and rather intimate relationship that acts as a rock in a time of stormy chaos. It is this holding ground that becomes the first real reference point to a clearer direction and a more hopeful future. That is not to undervalue the technical skills of the therapist but it is also not to make light of the benefits of listening, respect and mutual engagement.

Although the messages from disabled people are simple, putting them into practice requires change at all levels of therapy education, practice, management and policy. Finkelstein (1991) contends that workers in rehabilitation services should see themselves as a resource for disabled people and advocates a new professional group which he terms Professions Allied to the Community (Finkelstein 2004). Similarly, Stone (1999) argues that rehabilitation professionals should be allied to disabled people rather than allied to medicine. Disability is not usually high on the political agenda of health authorities and resources may be limited when compared with other areas of health and social care, but therapists do have agency to bring about change in their places of work. This will be discussed in the following chapters.

CONCLUSION

This chapter has highlighted the views and experiences of disabled people regarding health professionals and health care. Disabled people value the technical expertise of therapists, if used in a way that enhances their lifestyles, but focus more on their interpersonal qualities valuing warmth, realism, flexibility, genuineness, honesty, kindness and the ability to share power and to work in partnership. Without these qualities therapy interventions are unlikely to succeed for success is dependent on engaging with disabled people's ideas, feelings, aspirations, expectations and lifestyles and recognizing that they are 'experts' on disability in their own right.

Chapter **6**

The experiences of disabled health and caring professionals

In this chapter we aim to bring to the fore the experiences of disabled health and caring professionals and, in doing so, to question the assumption (often unspoken) that disabled people are patients and clients rather than people capable of dispensing professional services. Although it might be considered that health and caring professionals would be knowledgeable and understanding regarding disabled people and would welcome them as colleagues, there is considerable evidence to suggest that this is not always the case (Abberley 1995, French 2001, French & Swain 2001). This is part of a wider picture of discrimination against disabled people in all forms of employment (Burchardt 2000, 2005, Roulstone & Barnes 2005). Using the Labour Force Survey of 2004, Sapey & Hughes (2005) found that only 49% of disabled people of working age were employed compared with 81% of non-disabled people and that they were under-represented among managerial and professional occupations. Furthermore because disabled people are often discriminated against in education, their qualifications tend to be considerably lower which may hinder employment prospects (Sapey & Hughes 2005).

It is now recognized that unless the workforce of any society reflects the citizens it serves then inequalities and discrimination will remain and a large resource of talent will be lost: indeed this is sometimes put forward as the 'business case' for employing disabled people. Simkiss (2004:28), for instance, states that:

> Employers are beginning to realise that recruiting and retaining disabled people brings advantages to their business … a diverse workforce can reflect the customer base.

Over the past thirty years various equality laws have been passed, for example the Sex Discrimination Act (1975), the Race Relations Act (1976), the Disability Discrimination Act (1995) and the Human Rights Act (1998) in an attempt to combat discrimination and to regulate the number of women, people from ethnic minorities and disabled people in work, education and other areas of society. The Disability Discrimination Act (1995), in particular, is weak and is still being enacted. As recently as 2002, for instance, it was revised to make discrimination in education, which had hitherto been absent from the Act, illegal and in December 2006 a duty was placed on all public bodies including hospitals, universities and primary care trusts to promote disability equality (Byron et al 2005).

As well as the broad issue of equality in society, of which employment is an important part, it can also be argued that employing disabled people within the health and caring professions has the potential to improve client services.

French has researched visually impaired physiotherapists working within the NHS focusing on the barriers they experience and the strategies they use to overcome or minimize them (French 1990, 2001). Research on the experiences of disabled health and caring professionals is extremely sparse so this study will be utilized throughout the chapter to highlight important points.

Visually impaired people have been educated as physiotherapists in sizeable numbers over the course of the 20th century to the present day. There are approximately 250 visually impaired physiotherapists practicing in Britain (privately and in the NHS) including many who are totally blind (French 2001). Physiotherapy is not a profession which would immediately spring to mind as being suitable for visually impaired people: it requires competent mobility around busy wards, considerable paperwork and the use of sophisticated electromedical equipment. In recent years other difficulties have arisen including an increase in community work that involves travel and varying environments.

It is interesting to note that visually impaired people are educated as physiotherapists because of an historical accident rather than as the result of a planned strategy of inclusion. Physiotherapy evolved from massage that blind people traditionally practised. Up until 1916 they were educated in small numbers in ordinary schools of massage but, with the First World War and the large number of blinded servicemen, a special school of massage was opened by the National Institute for the Blind in London which, as the profession developed, became a school of physiotherapy. This segregated arrangement lasted until 1995. Visually impaired people are now integrated into mainstream physiotherapy courses within universities. With one or two minor exceptions they have followed the same syllabus as other physiotherapy students. This historical accident has an important lesson to teach in that disabled people can be very successful in professions that, on the surface, look unsuitable or even impossible (French 2001). Visually impaired people have achieved prominent positions within physiotherapy in a variety of roles including education and management.

WHY EMPLOY DISABLED HEALTH AND CARING PROFESSIONALS?

 Activity 6.1

THE BENEFITS OF EMPLOYING DISABLED THERAPISTS

On your own or with a colleague, write down any benefits you can think of for employing disabled people as therapists.

When you have done this read the quotations below, taken from interviews with visually impaired physiotherapists (from French 1990, with permission) and make a list of the advantages of being disabled in that role from the perspective of the physiotherapists themselves.

I understand mobility problems more than anything else – outdoor mobility problems that is. I've found myself recommending Dial-a-Ride to quite a few of my elderly patients recently. I know the difficulty of getting out and coping with awkward journeys. I know how it feels to me, so I can imagine how difficult it must be for them if their mobility is poor or their exercise tolerance is low.

(p. 2)

Our sensitivity to people is enhanced ... there are times when I feel slighted or embarrassed or frustrated. It's there all the time. This makes me much more conscious when someone comes to me with an arthritic knee, which I don't happen to have. I can understand the feelings they have when they can't get on the bus and the humiliation this causes them.

(p. 2)

Often they can relate to my disability with their own troubles – having to be dependent on others, having to ask people for help, things like that. They often say, 'You know all about this don't you?'

(p. 3)

I think it's easier for us to talk to someone with an ongoing problem ... I have quite a few MS patients. I never compare myself with them but when they say 'I don't want to use a stick' or 'I don't want to use a wheelchair', I tell them that I wouldn't use a white stick until I was in my late twenties and I found myself avoiding journeys because I would have to cross the road. I tell them that by getting the white stick out I am able to do any journey because I know someone will help me. I tell them that by using a prop you keep your independence. Most of them seem to accept what I am suggesting. Some have said, 'I see, I've never looked at it like that.' I emphasise that they are not giving in to the disease – they're accepting it, they're getting over it.

(p. 4–5)

I'm not put off by anyone's appearance, it cannot alter any way in which I think or feel about them.

(p. 6)

It makes you a much better listener ... because we don't use vision we really listen to what is being said. We assimilate it more and think more about what has been said.

(p. 4)

My patients find it helpful when they've been out of work for some time and I tell them about me being out of work for five years. I tell them that I reorganised my life and I'm doing all right ... A lot of them think it's the end of the world when they are about to lose their job because they've lost their leg or something ... I point out that it is possible to take a new path and be successful. They listen to me because there's a bit of fellow-feeling. I use it as a lever to show them they can cope.

(p. 5)

If you're treating a group of young blokes who have just had a meniscectomy and they're being a bit babyish and you come as a blind person, they think 'Goodness, that chap's working against the odds'. It changes them.

(p. 5)

I had a patient last week who referred his son. He said 'He's getting depressed about his back problem but when he sees you and how you're motivated he'll soon be all right.

(p. 5)

Were your ideas about the benefits of employing disabled therapists similar or different from those of the visually impaired physiotherapists? Do any of the points they raise surprise you and if so in what way? Do you think the same would apply to health and caring professionals with different impairments?

Many of these quotations focus on the empathy the visually impaired physiotherapists have for their patients. Issues that disabled people have in common with each other, regardless of their particular impairment, were mentioned. These included feelings of frustration and embarrassment and coping with the disabling environment, for example getting on and off buses and managing outdoor mobility. Similar points were made in an earlier study of disabled health and caring professionals (French 1988) where a deaf occupational therapist remarked 'They don't see me as a health professional who knows it all, who doesn't really understand, they see me as a disabled person' (1988:178) and a doctor said:

> Very many people have told me they can talk to me because I know what it feels like to have an illness. Once you get over that hump of being accepted (for training) in the first place, then you can use your disability.
>
> (French 1988:178)

The visually impaired physiotherapists felt that the social divide between themselves (as professionals) and their patients was reduced by disability. Patients recognized that the physiotherapists would be coping, or would have been through, similar experiences to themselves which could lead to 'a bit of fellow-feeling'. Similarly a blind social worker interviewed by French believed that needing help from clients was one of the advantages of being disabled in that it helped to equalize the relationship:

> I'm able to say to my clients, 'I'll help you but there are certain ways in which you are going to have to help me' and the client doesn't feel totally taken over or totally worthless.
>
> (French 1988:178)

Although excessive self-disclosure is inappropriate in any therapeutic relationship (Burnard 1992), the physiotherapists' carefully disclosed specific experiences – gaining independence by using a white stick, finding a new occupation after becoming disabled – help their patients view disability differently and behave towards it in a more optimistic and positive way. Their willingness to ask for help could also give a strong message that needing some assistance does not equate to inability or dependency.

The final three quotations suggest that the visually impaired physiotherapists may serve as role models for their patients and may help them to put their own condition or situation into perspective. Meeting other disabled people and seeing how they manage can be powerful but it can also be problematic. As one of the physiotherapists said, 'It can work two ways. If they see you coping it can encourage them or depress them. You've got to be very astute about which way they're going' (French 1990:5). A similar view was expressed by a prosthetist who had had an amputation himself. He reported that despite the benefit of shared experience, patients would sometimes say, 'If only I could walk like you' (French 1986:83) which made him very careful never to compare himself with his patients or expect them to cope in the same way. A doctor with multiple sclerosis who also took part in this study, viewed the advantages of being disabled in his role from a wide perspective (French 1988:179):

> MS has been something I've used. Having MS has been an added dimension in my training, in my understanding of people, and in the development of my expertise and skills.

The visually impaired physiotherapists also believed that the need for them to touch their patients more (for example when checking that an exercise was being performed correctly) was an advantage – touch, in itself, is well known to have therapeutic value (Vickers et al 2005). The idea that other skills, for example listening, may be developed more fully because of visual impairment were also mentioned by the physiotherapists.

There is no reason to suppose that a non-disabled health therapist would be incapable of understanding and helping patients in the ways described above or, indeed, that a disabled therapist would necessarily be skilled in this regard. However, the direct experience of disability that disabled health and caring professionals have is likely, on balance, to provide a richer and deeper understanding of disability provided that the uniqueness of every individual is kept centrally in mind. The presence of disabled people in the workforce, particularly if they are in sufficient numbers, is also likely to gradually change the prevailing occupational culture in the same way as an influx of women into traditional male occupations, such as medicine, is likely to do.

It is important that disabled health and caring professionals can choose the specialties in which they work and that they are not expected to work with disabled people or to be 'experts' in disability. The following quotations, from a social worker and a counsellor illustrate how this can happen:

> I wanted to get away from the feeling within me and within everybody else that all I could do was work with the blind.
>
> (French 1986:85)

> They always assumed I'd do disability counselling, they were hanging a label around my neck.
>
> (French 1986:85)

BARRIERS FACED BY DISABLED HEALTH AND CARING PROFESSIONALS

An important factor that hinders health and caring professionals in their ability to empathize and understand disabled people is the lack of emphasis on disability studies (the social, political and cultural analysis of disability) in the curriculum and the strong emphasis on medical conditions and impairments. Disability studies has been promoted largely by disabled activists and disabled academics from various disciplines, particularly sociology. Before the advent of disability studies much of the theoretical analysis of disability on which practice is based took place within medicine and psychology where the voices of disabled people themselves were rarely heard (Swain et al 2003). Levinson & Parritt (2005:120), talking about psychologists, state:

> There is already a large body of research, conducted by disabled people and organisations … of which the majority of psychologists in every field remain largely unaware to the detriment of their profession.

This situation is certainly true of physiotherapy and occupational therapy education where disability studies, if represented at all, is hidden within the social science curriculum that is itself small when compared with that of the 'hard' sciences. The lack of understanding of disability within the health and caring professions is illustrated in the following quotations that show how two doctors changed their views about disability when they became disabled themselves.

> Although I was a physician I was not informed by the perspective of disabled people … I was horrified by what I imagined to be the experiences of disabled people, which I encountered in my practice. Now, 15 years after becoming disabled, I find myself completely at home with the concept of effectively being me! … Now I know that my assessment of the potential quality of life for severely disabled people was clearly flawed.
>
> (Basnett 2001:453)

> As in so many areas of life, knowing how little you know is the important thing … The disability I know best is deafness. The profession I know best is medicine. So I accept that I have no idea of what life is like for, say, an accountant with cerebral palsy. But I do at least know what not to do if I meet such a person. I won't automatically assume that they can't do certain things – nor will I blithely reassure them that they can … Above all I will let them tell me how it is.
>
> (Kvalsing 2003:63)

Activity 6.2

DIFFICULTIES WHICH MAY BE FACED BY DISABLED THERAPISTS

On your own or with a colleague, make a list of all the reasons you can think of why disabled people may find it problematic to work as health and caring professionals or to enter these professions.

The lack of interest in understanding disability from the perspective of disabled people has serious repercussions in the health and caring professions that may be difficult to face. As Byron et al (2005:12) state:

> For professions that consider themselves founded on principles of caring and service, it is uncomfortable to have to acknowledge the reality that healthcare is endemically disablist.

You may have come up with some of the following reasons:

- Inability to cope with some or all aspects of the job because of impairment.
- Inaccessible equipment.
- Health and safety regulations.
- Rigid work schedules and routines.
- Prejudice and discrimination from managers, colleagues, professional bodies and assessors.
- Objections from patients and clients.
- Perceptions of disabled people as recipients of care rather than caregivers.
- Inaccessible buildings.
- Inaccessible transport.
- Lack of educational opportunities.
- The need to work fast and flexibly.

Although there may, on occasions, be a reason to deny a disabled person a specific type of employment (a blind person would be unsuitable as a surgeon, for example), the reasoning behind the rejection of disabled people in the workforce, including the health and caring professions, is usually due to ignorance, prejudice and institutional discrimination (Sapey & Hughes 2005). It is also the case that disabled people, being experts on their own capabilities, are very unlikely to put themselves forward for employment they cannot undertake successfully.

The difficulty of viewing disabled people in the role of health or caring professionals, by those already in the professions, is highlighted by Levinson & Parritt (2005:114) who contend that 'The professional role of a disabled colleague clashes with stereotypes of disability which are firmly linked to patients'. They go on to recount how the strength of this stereotype can lead to embarrassing situations where receptionists and others firmly believe that disabled professionals are patients. Similar behaviour was noted by Kerr (1977:48) nearly thirty years ago:

> I have been wheeling along to treatment settings in various parts of the country attending to my business as a clinical psychologist, when an attendant or nurse would bustle alongside me and challengingly or sarcastically say, 'Hey, where do you think you're going?' On more than one occasion my wheelchair has been hi-jacked by an attendant who, without comment, wheeled me into the dining room of the institution.

Most of the overt justification for the exclusion of disabled people from the health and caring professions is in terms of disabled people themselves; their presumed inability to cope, the adverse effects they may have on patients and clients, and the assumption of proneness to accidents (French 1994b, French 2001). Stannett (2005) reports, for example, that he was compelled to leave a psychology course that required clinical work for one that did not on account of the attitudes of professionals towards his speech impairment. Sutherland (1981:41) believes that these attitudes are so ingrained that they are not even questioned:

> When we are discriminated against for such reasons the people who find us unsuitable for the job or training course that we have applied for do so in good faith, they think that they have made a fair decision and would deny that any unfair discrimination has taken place … they judge us as unsuitable because that is really how we look to them.

Such attitudes are likely to have a damaging effect on disabled people who are trying to find their place in the world of work. This is illustrated by Boazman who qualified as a counsellor after a stroke that left her aphasic. She relates how, after three years of training, one of her assessors expressed strong reservations about her ability to work as a counsellor and the devastating effect that this had on her (Boazman 1999:19–20):

> The emotional damage that this report had on me was catastrophic … my confidence was destroyed from that moment on … I began to doubt my own ability and thought long and hard about my ability to become a counsellor. For a while I had certainly lost my sense of identity and my self image was at an all time low.

Sivanesan (2003:569), a visually impaired occupational therapist, relates similar attitudes from professionals:

> I entered the field of occupational therapy fully aware that my visual impairment would make the whole experience more challenging. However, I did not foresee other people's reactions to my disability. I would often encounter concerns about my ability to succeed in my chosen profession.

Levinson & Parritt (2005:115) state that:

> It is an uncomfortable experience to be told that your very presence may be awkward for other people. And to hear misgivings about your competence to deal with patients may be very undermining. There is a strong element of stereotyping underlying this response, together with a subtle form of rejection. These colleagues are asking how a patient can be a provider of therapy.

Green (2005:2), a deaf physiotherapy student, explains the difference it can make when clinicians have positive attitudes:

> My confidence slowly came up as I had extremely good clinicians who never assumed anything of me, and asked me questions about my deafness which I found helped our working relationship … What amused me this year, along with the second year, is that the first strength that my clinicians wrote down on my marking form was communication.

However, on another placement a clinician criticized the way she preferred to learn from books rather than from group work which resulted in 'anger and low confidence' (Green 2005:3). Group interaction is, of course, particularly difficult for deaf people to manage unless careful adjustments are made.

Negative attitudes are sometimes rationalized and disguised as concern, emphasizing that disabled people may damage themselves or others by undertaking such demanding work. Alan Dudley, a blind social worker we interviewed said:

> There were concerns about situations they were putting me in, whether there were dangers to me and whether I was at risk. There were concerns about how I perceive situations when I have no sight. Would I pick up nuances and subtleties? Would I be able to describe situations accurately because of that? Practical things like would I be able to get to the houses and so forth … Situations like, how would I deal with it if I got threatened or even attacked and would they somehow be to blame for that?
>
> (French et al 1997:40)

Such rationalizations have almost certainly been fuelled by health and safety legislation and fears of litigation (Willcocks et al 1998).

Levinson & Parritt (2005) highlight various psychological mechanisms which operate towards disabled people both when they seek employment and once they are employed. Disability may, for instance, be denied in order to reduce the role confusion generated by disabled health and caring professionals (who are perceived as patients and clients), especially when disabled people are in positions of power and control. Carole Pound (2004:33), a disabled speech and language therapist, comments on the 'divided identity' she experiences:

> I am struggling to interact with you simultaneously as Carole the speech and language therapist and Carole the 'patient', the person on the other side of the rehabilitation divide. This divided identity is a fascinating issue. Two selves so clearly related and yet so carefully circumscribed and kept distinct.

The fear and anxiety surrounding the employment of disabled people as health and caring professionals may be projected onto patients and clients leading non-disabled professionals to believe that patients are worried about being treated by a disabled person. Excessive anxiety from colleagues can also stifle the autonomy of disabled colleagues and render professional relationships unequal.

Goffman (1963), in his discourse on stigma, notes that those closely associated with disabled people are subject to negative stereotyping where they become 'tarred with the same brush' as disabled people. This he refers to as a 'courtesy stigma'. Thus it may be felt that the prestige or power of a profession is reduced by the presence of disabled colleagues. Sutherland (1981:40) states that, 'Since the job for which the person is applying would confer a recognition of equality, they tend not to get it, they are judged unsuitable'. If disabled professionals are viewed as clients, or inferior to non-disabled people, this may also affect the self-esteem of non-disabled professionals. This was highlighted by a visually impaired physiotherapist who said:

> Often there is an air of 'I feel very proud of this profession, and I do very complicated things, so how on earth can someone without sight do it too? … it deflates their ego, it's an imperious attitude, a sense of jealousy. I found it when I was a superintendent and someone said to me 'this is an easy job, the department runs itself'.
> (French 2001:154)

Attitudes such as this may also impact on promotion.

Another important issue when considering the employment of disabled people as health and caring professionals is the criteria on which they are judged to be suitable. Until recent times people with a wide range of impairments and other characteristics were barred from becoming health and caring professionals and attitudes towards their recruitment were poor. French (1987) found, for example, that 158 (76%) of a sample of 209 physiotherapists believed that someone with restricted shoulder movement was unsuitable for employment as a physiotherapist and 114 (54%) thought that deaf people were unsuitable. Sapey & Hughes believe that professional bodies need to demonstrate that the standards they impose can be objectively justified and do not amount to discrimination. This applies both to assessment and recruitment. They state (2005: 298–299):

> … the bodies responsible for both reviewing and applying the standards will in most cases be closely associated with occupations that have shown themselves to be less than responsive to the challenge of the disabled people's movement … to achieve any degree of equality in either the review or assessment of competence standards, it will be necessary for qualification bodies to think in revolutionary ways about the standards they are charged with upholding.

OVERCOMING BARRIERS

◆ *Activity 6.3*

BARRIERS TO PRACTICE FOR DISABLED THERAPISTS

Read the following quotations from visually impaired physiotherapists (from French 2001, with permission) and write a few sentences about the barrier or barriers each of the physiotherapists highlight. Then go back to the list you made in Activity 6.2 and see how many of the barriers you identified are similar. How far are they to do with impairment? What mechanisms could be put in place to overcome or minimize the barriers experienced?

Definitely it's easier to work in the out-patient department than struggle round the wards trying to find the patients ... I haven't got enough sight to recognise a patient by any sort of facial feature unless I've seen them for a great many days. In most wards patients are moved around, as they become less acutely ill they're shunted up the ward ... I'd go to the old bed first, and the patient had gone and then I'd have to start hunting for him so that was by far the worst thing. And I suppose the next difficult aspect was the anxiety about how many bottles, tubes and drips were likely to be attached to the patient. I would go very slowly and cautiously so as never to knock anything over, and luckily I never did, but that was an anxiety. And of course if the lighting wasn't very good then that added to all the problems.
(p. 129–130)

There's some stuff around nowadays that is not easy to use. I bung bits of 'high-mark' (a tactile marking substance) on, which does work on the whole.

One interferential machine we've got is not easy to use. In fact as a totally blind person, or a non-display reading person, you wouldn't be able to use it. But there is an older one that I can use ... You can still find stuff but you have to look around ... They're using more visual displays and it's all computerised, it's very flat, you don't have the landmarks that you used to have, there's the touch-sensitive keyboard thing. It's the way everything has gone, if you look throughout domestic appliances it's the same.

(p. 120)

I have to go everywhere by bus. The problem is I have to deliver frames, so I sometimes have to get on a bus with a walking frame ... I try and avoid it when the kids are going to school, or coming home from school, or in the rush hour ... I've managed it so far. If I get really desperate, like if I have a really big piece of equipment to take, then I'll tell the manager and she'll arrange for me to go round in a cab and drop it off.

(p. 118)

I've worked in some very difficult situations with some very autocratic doctors and at team meetings it's a problem of picking up their non-verbal communication, when they're getting angry and things. To a certain extent it affected my ability to handle difficult situations, you know, knowing when it might be best to say nothing.

(p. 137)

One course I went on recently, the chap went through it at such a rate of knots that I did miss out quite a bit. As a senior you are expected to do your part in the teaching and if you say, 'I don't feel happy to teach that because I didn't grasp it all' it reflects back on you. You're the one that looks inadequate. People have never understood.

(p. 95)

I'm a registered blind person but they haven't got a clue ... If I stay in one building I'm fine, it's only when I go over to G ... that I get really lost ... and one of the physios says, 'So you're not talking to me today!' because I've walked right past them ... and I've worked with them for years; oh dear! ... I just say 'I didn't see you' but they don't seem to learn.

(p. 140)

I was relocated to another hospital which was extremely difficult for me to get to from home. It required catching three buses. So I actually had to take out a grievance with the Trust about it ... the Access to Work people supported me partially to help me with taxi fares home. I walked in the morning, and it was over three miles, but I got a taxi home in the evening.

(p. 118)

I didn't like the weekends because you had to go on to wards that you weren't familiar with and you had to rely so much on your echo location (the detection of objects through sound) for getting around. You can echo locate in familiar surroundings very quickly but when you go to unfamiliar ones you have to go a lot more slowly and of course you're that much more tense. The mental exhaustion of concentration in unfamiliar surroundings is quite tiresome.

(p. 129)

Many of the problems the physiotherapists experienced concerned environmental and structural barriers. In the past, visually impaired physiotherapists, and other disabled employees, had to rely on their own tenacity and the goodwill of colleagues and managers to circumvent or manage these problems but now, with the Disability Discrimination Act (1995) in place, the need for support at work, if required, and the need to work in a different way from that of colleagues has become a right, although the Disability Discrimination Act (1995) remains weak. Under the Access to Work scheme (which existed in a very modified form for many years before the Disability Discrimination Act was passed), accessible technology may be supplied as well as help with transport and personal assistants who, for example, can help with administration. Although such assistance does not solve all the problems some of the physiotherapists spoke enthusiastically about it. This is illustrated in the following quotations:

> My world changed the day I got a computer. Really, I can't tell you, it's the most revolutionary thing that has happened to me since I've been a physio ... I've always had problems with notes, every job I've ever been in nobody could read my hand-writing. I used to use a typewriter and then I applied to get a computer from the Access to Work scheme and I got given some training and, believe me, it's the best thing that ever happened to me ... I flash it all up on the screen, all my patients' notes, current and from years gone by, large as I want. I can also print things out in large print so I can read it back.
>
> (French 2001:124–125)

> The Trust has put at my disposal a car which I use for business mileage ... it does mean that if I have to go to say ... Leeds to sit on the NHS Equal Opportunities Working Party ... the assistant actually drives me there.
>
> (French 2001:120)

Although the attitudes and behaviour of colleagues was cited as a problem by some of the physiotherapists, many others had had positive experiences and the help of colleagues was regarded as essential for success in their professional role. One of the physiotherapists explained how colleagues assisted him with paper work which he regarded as a better solution than using technology (French 2001:128):

> I'm lucky that the helpers, and all the staff generally, help with all the extra bits of paper that are around. The truth of the matter is that, as a blind person, you could get involved in form filling by

putting it on the computer, but what the hell's the point because it's going to take an awful lot of time.

Another physiotherapist, who was near to retirement, spoke of the help she had received from her manager (French 2001:128–129):

> I find that even though she's very high-powered, she's eager to get my ability to cope with the computer sorted out and the secretary to help me if necessary. I said I would pay for some extra secretarial help myself but she said 'no, no, we'll sort is out another way'.

The exchange of help between colleagues at work is, of course, commonplace and it is likely that the visually impaired physiotherapists reciprocated the help they received in other ways.

Although one of the major concerns expressed about the employment of disabled health and caring professionals is the effect they may have on patients, it is extremely rare for disabled health and caring professionals to have problems in this regard. Levinson & Parritt (2005:115) state:

> On the whole we can report favourably on our interactions with patients and clients as neither of us have encountered any overt reactions … Almost without exception, we have found that provided patients/clients perceived that they were receiving adequate attention to their problems, and that the interaction and therapy appeared to benefit them, so they were apparently unconcerned about disability.

Many of the visually impaired physiotherapists regarded the helpfulness of patients as a major strategy in their ability to succeed. This is illustrated in the following quotations:

> I didn't need to ask for help in the wards I worked on every day because once the patients knew who you were they couldn't wait to shout 'Stop, there's a table!' You'd say 'Where's Mr. Brown?' and they'd say 'Hang on, I'll go and look for him'. The patients were my first ally.
>
> (French 2001:135)

> They would assist you in locating them themselves by shouting out 'Ere I am' and they would ensure that you didn't clobber into something on your way out of the ward by instructing you verbally or, if they were fit enough, actually escorting you out. I always found the patients very helpful if they were well enough to be so.
>
> (French 2001:136)

> They're very good, very accepting, not worried at all about having a totally blind physio work with them. One or two queries about

whether I'd be able to manage this or that, but literally only one or two over the whole of the years I've been working which is not bad going. They've been very friendly and very chatty and obviously quite interested as well.

(French 2001:136)

This study of visually impaired physiotherapists indicates that barrier removal can be very complex. Despite sophisticated computer equipment, for example, most of the physiotherapists felt that it took them considerably more time to successfully hold down their jobs. Reliance on cognitive strategies was said to be exhausting and most people were motivated to change the environment rather than attempt to change themselves. There was considerable difference regarding the impact of barriers according to the level of the physiotherapist's sight. Blind physiotherapists, for example, were more likely to be offered help but many tasks were more difficult for them than those with some sight, for example coping in strange environments. People also used different methods to minimize barriers, for example audiotape, large print, Braille or a combination of these were used to access written information.

Although there was considerable agreement among the physiotherapists with regard to barriers and coping strategies, it was also clear from this study that barriers are perceived, appraised, experienced and acted upon differently. Both contextual factors (for example position in the hierarchy) and individual factors (confidence and assertion) can modify barriers and how they are dealt with.

The physiotherapists were prepared to cope with difficult barriers in order to satisfy their own goals and aspirations. People did not necessarily work in areas where lack of sight was less of a problem although some people did go into private practice in order to create their own environment. Reasons such as 'believing in the NHS', 'not being a businessperson', 'needing the stimulation of other people' or being interested in a particular clinical area dissuaded many of the physiotherapists from private practice or taking an easier option. A totally blind physiotherapist, for example, spoke enthusiastically of community work since the institution for people with learning difficulties where she previously worked had closed (French 2001:150):

It's very stimulating because you come into contact with a lot of different people. Since we came out of L (the institution) we've had referrals from people who have never had treatment before … so we've met an awful lot more families and carers and I find that keeping all the balls going in the air at once is really stimulating.

The physiotherapists found that work had become easier in some ways, for example less overt discrimination, but had become harder in other ways, for example increased community work, increased paperwork, a faster turnover of patients and an increased pace of work. Overall the physiotherapists felt that work had become more difficult despite the introduction of equal opportunity policies and the Disability Discrimination Act (1995).

SUPPORTING DISABLED HEALTH AND CARING PROFESSIONALS

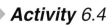

Activity 6.4

HOW MAY COLLEAGUES HELP?

On your own or with a colleague make a list of the things you could do to assist disabled colleagues at work. Remember that they will be fully competent to undertake the work although they may need to do things in a different way.

In our view the most important thing you can do is to ask the disabled person if any help is required and precisely how you can help. This goes back to the quotation by Kvalsing (2003:63), the disabled doctor, who said 'As in so many areas of life, knowing how little you know is the important thing'. Health and caring professionals are socialized into the role of 'expert' which can make it difficult to learn from disabled people. This is, however, essential (with patients and clients as well as colleagues) if the relationship is to be successful. It is also important that the disabled person is treated as an individual and not compared with similar people you may have met. Impairment is only one facet of the entire person and the way people deal with it, as well as the way they appraise and cope with the barriers they encounter, will depend on many factors including their personality, past experience and the context they are in.

It is important too that any help you give is consistent, for example facing a deaf colleague when you talk or ensuring that a colleague who uses a wheelchair is not obstructed by obstacles. It can be exhausting for disabled people to contend with barriers and barrier removal on their own and non-disabled allies are almost always welcomed in the struggle to achieve an accessible environment. As noted above, it is a normal aspect of working life that colleagues help each other. Although the assistance needed by disabled colleagues may be different it is unlikely to be any more time consuming and, as disabled people have as many skills and talents as anyone else, they will be able to return the help in full.

It should be remembered that under the Disability Discrimination Act (1995) disabled employees are entitled to work in a non-disabling environment on equal terms with their colleagues. Disabled health and caring professionals should not be expected to 'fit in' and the managers of organizations in which they work have many responsibilities in terms of, for example, staff education and accessible buildings and equipment to ensure that disabled people can fulfil their role. None of this is to minimize, however, the importance of consideration, practical help and a positive attitude from colleagues on a day-to-day basis.

CONCLUSION

In this chapter we have highlighted the need of professions such as occupational therapy and physiotherapy to recruit more disabled people into their ranks. This, we believe, will benefit the professions in terms of their representation that, in turn, has the potential to enhance practice. Disabled people have a wealth of experience and knowledge of disability that the health and caring professions need to tap for the benefit of disabled people and themselves.

Chapter 7

Controlling services

This chapter concerns the role of health professionals in the lives of disabled people. As we discussed in Chapter 5, although some disabled people have found the interventions of professionals and professional services helpful, others have been critical of the control professionals have over their lives and the restrictive nature of the services they provide (French 2004). This situation has led disabled people to create their own innovative services and to press for legislation that gives them greater control over those provided by statutory bodies (Barnes & Mercer 2006).

In this chapter we focus directly on power relationships in providing services, as this issue manifests itself in many guises. First we examine the professional side of the relationship and, in particular, question the dominant, traditional views of what it means to be a professional. We then turn the tables and explore the provision of services by disabled people themselves and the consequent relationship with professionals.

PROFESSIONALS IN CONTROL

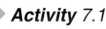

Activity 7.1

WHAT IS A PROFESSION?

'Profession' and 'professional' are not easy terms to define. Spend a few minutes jotting down your own definition of a profession and a professional worker.

The terms 'profession' and 'professional' are used in a variety of ways. We may comment that the builder has done a 'professional' job, meaning that the job is done well, or that the shop assistant behaved 'professionally' when dealing with an awkward customer. When asked to name which occupations are professions, however, most people would not opt for builder or shop assistant but would probably choose doctor or lawyer, though some may mention teacher, nurse, therapist or social worker. At its simplest level a profession can be defined as a particular type of occupation.

One way of defining whether or not an occupation is a profession is provided by the 'trait' approach or 'trait' model (Abbott & Meerabeau 1998). With this model, professions are defined in terms of distinct traits or characteristics.

Activity 7.2

THE TRAIT MODEL OF PROFESSIONALISM

Make a list of any traits or characteristics that, in your view, define the meaning of 'profession' and 'professional'. In order to do this, think about your own work as an occupational therapist or physiotherapist and what distinguishes your work from that of a non-professional worker.

Many lists of traits that are said to define professions have been drawn up, although few professions aspire to them all (Hugman 1991). You may have written down some of the following traits or characteristics of the physiotherapy and occupational therapy professions:

- The skills within occupational therapy and physiotherapy are based upon theoretical knowledge.
- The work carries responsibility and is not routine. It often involves analysis and interpretation.
- The work is orientated to public service and is highly skilled.

Physiotherapists and occupational therapists:

- are trustworthy
- have an organized professional body which regulates training and selects, assesses, safeguards and controls its members
- adhere to a professional code of conduct through a code of ethics
- have the power to make autonomous decisions

- have a monopoly over a certain area of work usually through legislation and registration
- are consulted (for example by government), and have an influence, on policy.

According to the trait model professionals are characterized by trust, respect, knowledge and the belief that they work for the benefit of their clients. Professionals are rewarded by autonomy, high status, power, control and often high pay (Waterfield 2004).

Medicine, divinity and law are frequently cited as 'pure' professions whereas occupations that are deemed to have gone some way to acquiring these traits are referred to as semi-professions. Semi-professions include nursing, social work, physiotherapy, occupational therapy and teaching. It has been difficult for some of these groups to professionalize fully because of the control of the medical profession over them. This is reflected in the terms 'paramedical professions' and 'professions supplementary to medicine'.

The specialist knowledge of professionals forms the foundation for developing philosophies, values and systems of work. Expert knowledge is thought to be essential if professionals are to be autonomous, self-regulating and trustworthy. Those occupations aspiring to become professions attempt to define their own body of knowledge and to separate it from 'lay' knowledge and the knowledge of other professions. In doing so they lengthen the period of training required, making it more specialized, and undertake research (Fulcher & Scott 1999). Many occupations, such as teaching, nursing, physiotherapy and occupational therapy, have moved into the university sector over the past 25 years where these aims can be pursued. Talking of physiotherapy, Waterfield (2004:191–192) states:

> ... physiotherapy has tried to mould its own professional development in fields such as postgraduate education, research and titled roles, to achieve professional recognition and possibly to achieve a similar status to that of medicine.

Semi-professions in the health sector have, however, lacked their own theoretical base and have tended to rely heavily on that of the powerful medical profession for their knowledge. The fact that the paramedical professions are dominated by women whereas the medical profession, and other 'pure' professions like law, are dominated by men, has also been significant in slowing down professionalization because of gender inequality. It is the case, however, that occupations like physiotherapy and occupational therapy, though limited by the control exerted by the

medical profession, have also gained status through their close association with it.

As well as the process of professionalization, it is also possible for de-
professionalization to occur as attitudes, values and practices within
society change. Doctors, for example, are less autonomous than they
once were, they more often work in multidisciplinary teams than they
did in the past and are more accountable to managers and patient groups
(Tovey 2000). Nurses, on the other hand, have increased their autonomy
by, for example, undertaking some practices, such as prescribing drugs,
that were once the province of the medical profession (Wilson 2000).

I (Sally) have seen many changes within the physiotherapy profession
which have led to a higher level of professionalization. When I qualified
as a physiotherapist in 1972 we were not permitted to treat patients
unless they were referred to us by a hospital consultant and we were
compelled to carry out the treatment that he or she (nearly always he)
prescribed. Over the years, however, physiotherapists have gained the
autonomy to decide upon treatments themselves and to treat patients
who are referred by nurses and other therapists. Another change
involves the education of physiotherapists. Until the early 1980s there
were no degree courses for physiotherapists but it is now an all-degree
profession with a strong emphasis on research which is, nonetheless, still
in its infancy. Physiotherapy education has moved from small colleges
situated in the grounds of NHS hospitals to universities, and Masters
degree courses have been developed. These changes are mirrored in
other professions such as nursing and occupational therapy. In a few universities, for example the University of Southampton, physiotherapists
and occupational therapists are being educated together, at least in part,
which gives more opportunity for co-operation.

So far in this chapter professions have been portrayed as learned occupational groups who are devoted to the pursuit of knowledge and the
welfare of their patients and clients. Professions and professionals have,
however, come under criticism from many groups including sociologists,
feminists, politicians and, as we saw in Chapter 5, disabled people.

◆ *Activity 7.3*

CRITICISMS OF THE TRAIT MODEL

Write down any reservations you have about professions or the role of
professionals and any scepticism you feel about the way professions
have been portrayed so far in this chapter. It may help you to think about

times when you have used the services of professionals yourself or in your own work as a professional. You may also like to think about some of the criticisms of health professionals that disabled people made in Chapter 5 or the experiences of disabled health professionals in Chapter 6.

Some of your reservations may have centred around ideas that professions and professionals are:

- controlling
- distant
- privileged
- self-interested
- domineering
- gatekeepers
- disempowering in their role as 'definers' of problems and their role in 'professionalizing' everyday knowledge and 'medicalizing' life.

This alternative view of professionals is portrayed within the 'power' model where the claims of professionals, for example expert knowledge and altruistic motives, are viewed as little more than rhetoric to justify occupational autonomy, privilege and self-interest. Whalley Hammell (2006:149) believes, for instance, that rehabilitation:

> … is a system which rehabilitation practitioners have largely failed to challenge because they are the beneficiaries of a status quo that affords them social status, prestige and power over those who must use their services.

It has been claimed that ideologies of professionalism justify, legitimate and privilege professional knowledge although, in reality, a great deal of this knowledge falls far short of proved and tested theory (Hugman 1991). It is stated by the Chartered Society of Physiotherapy (2002:26), for example, that 'Many modalities in physiotherapy, although appearing to have a beneficial effect, have not been evaluated or researched'.

According to this model, skills are mystified (through jargon, for example) to widen the gap between professionals and their clients and to increase the dependency of those who seek professional advice (Hugman 1991). Sociologists such as Illich et al (1977) and McKnight (1995) regard professions as disabling as they diminish people's ability to look after themselves, and feminists have spoken about the patriarchal nature of the professions where high-ranking doctors and lawyers, for instance, tend to be white, male and with 'social connections'. As Davies (1998:193) states:

> We need to recognise the cloak of professionalism for the outdated and male-tailored garment that it is. Nineteenth century ideas about what it was to be a responsible gentleman, to work hard to cultivate, not land but knowledge, and to apply it from a lofty and distant class position needs serious amendment in the society of today.

Many people now believe that, to be effective, the composition of professions should reflect the communities that they serve (Waterfield 2004).

In recent times professions and professionals have also been challenged by government who have attacked their exclusivity by introducing a 'market economy' into health and social care (Nettleton 1998) (see Ch. 3). Recent scandals, such as that of Dr Shipman who was convicted of murdering 15 of his patients, have underlined the need for regulation and greater accountability on the part of professionals. There has been a lessening of trust of professionals which is reflected in greater control of their activities. The Health Professions Council, for example, now makes it mandatory for physiotherapists and occupational therapists to show evidence of continuing professional development in order to maintain their NHS registration. Government policy, such as the NHS and Community Care Act (1990), the Health and Social Care Act (2001) and the National Health Service Reform and Health Care Professions Act (2002), also promote 'user involvement' in policy and practice although it has been argued that this is patchy and often tokenistic (French & Swain in press). Finlay (2000b:74) writes:

> ... the place of the profession in modern society has become a much explored area of discussion and research. Some scholars and commentators have been critical of professionals' power and how they maintain their advantage in society. Others suggest that professionals are losing their hold in the face of marketisation, new regulations and consumer power.

Professionals have also been accused of engaging in 'social closure' whereby they seek to maximize their rewards and status by restricting the opportunities of others, policing their own activities and monopolizing a particular social and economic niche (Abbott & Meerabeau 1998). Complementary and alternative practitioners are, for example, generally debarred from working within the NHS though there are many exceptions and little guidance from central government on the extent of their inclusion (Heller 2005). It is the case, however, that if an unorthodox treatment become sufficiently popular to pose a threat, traditional practitioners tend to master it and practise it themselves. Physiotherapists, for example, now practise manipulation and acupuncture within the NHS whereas such practices, and any contact with alternative practitioners, were strongly discouraged when I (Sally) was a young physiotherapist. Richman (1987:227) contends that '… what is considered alternative medicine is the product of the powerful definers, who support establishment medicine'. In recent years most professions have been put under pressure (by the Disability Discrimination Act 1995, for instance) to instigate 'equal opportunity' policies and not to exclude people from entering the professions on the grounds of, for instance, ethnicity, gender and disability.

A further view of professionals is that they are 'agents of social control', that is people who control and stabilize society on behalf of the state by individualizing social problems. This is achieved by focusing on the individual rather than dealing with social and environmental factors, like poor housing and lack of education, that promote inequalities in health, and social problems such as drug abuse and crime. Thus a doctor may legitimate a few days' absence from work or recommend a counsellor for a stressed employee, rather than exploring the social, environmental and organizational origins of the stress. In this way the status quo, and the interests of powerful groups within society, are maintained (French & Swain 2001). As Kielhofner (2004:241) states '… therapy aims to eliminate client characteristics and traits that threaten the legitimacy of mainstream values, ideals, practices and rules'. Hugman (1991) points out that the trait model ignores the issue of power in the success of an occupation gaining professional status. The medical profession, for example, already had considerable power when negotiating its position with the state in the 19th century (Brunton 2004) and when the NHS was introduced in 1948 (Ham 1999).

Professional codes of ethics have also been criticized for having as much to do with professional etiquette and protectionism as with morality. In the publication *Rules of Professional Conduct* by the Chartered Society of Physiotherapy (2002:6), for example, it states that 'Chartered physiotherapists shall adhere at all times to personal and professional standards which reflect credit on the profession' and that colleagues should not be criticized except in a court of law. Homan (1991:3) concludes that '… ethical principles are established on the basis of a considerable measure of professional self-interest' and Whalley Hammell (2006:162–163) contends that '… rehabilitation professionals have given little attention to the political and ethical implications of serving two masters – the system in which they are employed and their clients'.

As people have become better educated and have greater access to information and opinion via television, radio and the Internet, professional knowledge is being increasingly challenged and deference towards professionals has diminished. Professional knowledge is no longer thought to be absolute but instead to reflect the attitudes and values of the profession, and to be just one point of view among many (Lee-Treweek 2005).

Activity 7.4

PHYSIOTHERAPY AND OCCUPATIONAL THERAPY – WHICH MODEL?

As you have seen, the trait model portrays professionals in a very positive light whereas the power model is more sceptical. You do not, of course, have to think in terms of 'either/or'. You may think, for instance, that therapists are altruistic but that they are also concerned with their professional status. You may believe that the 'social control' function of professions is a valuable one or that, in reality, therapists have little power in the face of governmental control. You may believe that 'social closure' is a thing of the past or that professions are still too selective in whom they recruit. Jot down your thoughts and feelings and, if possible, discuss them with a colleague or somebody outside your profession.

DISABLED PEOPLE IN CONTROL

In this section of the chapter we will be discussing Centres for Independent (or Integrated) Living (CILs) which disabled people have developed for themselves. Hasler (2006:286) defines a CIL as '… an organisation controlled by disabled people, providing support for independent living'.

As discussed in Chapter 5, it is important to understand that when disabled people talk of 'independence' they are not talking about the ability to care for themselves in a narrow, physical sense but the ability to take control of their lives. As Mason (2000:66) states:

> We know that we have to gain control over our lives even when we need help from others to function. Unless we do this, we can never make a real contribution to society because our own thoughts will never be expressed through our actions, only those of other people, our 'carers' … Therefore we redefine 'independence' to mean having control over your life, not 'doing things without help'.

An official definition of independent living by the Disability Rights Commission (2005:1) mirrors that of Mason:

> Independent living for disabled people ... means having the same choice, control and freedom as other citizens at home, work, in education and as equal citizens.

Our aim in this section of the chapter is to highlight the ways in which services run by disabled people differ from those of statutory and voluntary services in what they offer, how the service is offered and the underlying ethos and philosophy. We hope that this will provide a concrete example of how the social model of disability (discussed in Ch. 2) can be put into practice in the context of services. It should be noted that professional workers, particularly social workers and occupational therapists, have on occasions been employed by disabled people in CILs and that the services provided can, on the surface at least, appear quite similar to the services that the health and caring professions provide.

Centres for Independent Living

Centres for Independent Living in Britain took their inspiration and impetus from CILs in the USA. The first CIL was opened in Berkeley, California in 1973 and there are now 300 similar centres throughout the USA (Charlton 2000). Centres for Independent Living have been established in most countries of the Western world and in a few countries of the majority world, for example Brazil and Zimbabwe (Oliver & Barnes 1998). Barnes & Mercer (2006:77) outline the history of CILs in Britain:

> Initially, in the early 1980s, user-controlled organisations were developed by groups of disabled people leaving residential care who were seeking practical solutions to overcome the absence of statutory or voluntary agency support for independent living in the community. These included Britain's first two Centres for Independent/ Integrated Living (CILs) in Hampshire and Derbyshire.

In Britain most CILs are linked, to some degree, with statutory and voluntary services and usually rely on them for part of their funding.

Centres for Independent Living are run *by* disabled people *for* disabled people although non-disabled allies and supporters are usually welcome. The centres provide many services including peer counselling, advocacy, maintenance of equipment, transport, training in independent living skills, housing, mentoring, attendant services and disability equality training, including training of the trainers. Some provide extensive databases on issues relevant to disabled people, such as accessible holiday venues, and undertake research. They also lobby members of parliament and help other groups of disabled people to organize democratically.

Their premises and information are as accessible to disabled people as possible with, for example, induction loops and information in Braille. However, accessibility is sometimes compromised by lack of funding, for example it may be difficult to obtain fully accessible premises in a convenient central location (Barnes & Mercer 2006).

Activity 7.5

THE PHILOSOPHY AND SERVICES OF CENTRES FOR INDEPENDENT LIVING

Read the following account of the Southampton Centre for Independent Living (SCIL). Make a list of the ways in which the services that are offered differ from those typically provided by statutory services and note the ways in which they are similar?

Southampton Centre for Independent Living (SCIL)

The SCIL was founded in 1984 by a group of disabled people. In the early days of the organization it was run by volunteers, but by 2004 it had 14 full- and part-time employees and an annual income of £565 000. The organization has a large group of volunteers and an active management committee. Its main sources of income are from local authorities and the National Lottery Charities Board. The organization has no core funding and is, therefore, dependent on raising money from its own projects. Such money is raised from various activities including disability equality training and consultancy.

The aims of the organization are:

- to provide a means by which disabled people may take control over their own lives, achieve full participation in all spheres of society and effect change in how they are viewed and treated
- to provide encouragement, assistance, advice, support and facilities to individuals and groups wishing to live independently
- to raise the expectations of disabled people, individually and collectively, and ensure their voice is heard (SCIL 2005:18).

The work of the SCIL is based around 12 basic needs which have been identified by disabled people. These are for:

1. an accessible environment
2. aids and equipment

3. personal assistance
4. an adequate income
5. advocacy and self-advocacy
6. counselling
7. accessible public transport
8. accessible/adapted housing
9. inclusive education and training opportunities
10. equal opportunities for employment
11. appropriate and accessible information
12. appropriate and accessible health care.

The SCIL works in all of these areas, either directly or by collaborating with other organizations such as the Eastleigh Advocacy Service which works with people with learning difficulties. The SCIL shares premises with the Disability Advice and Information Network which enables easy communication and collaboration between them. In 2004–2005 its funded projects were: to supply information and support to disabled people receiving direct payments; to provide disability equality training in a wide range of organizations; to assist disabled people in recruiting and employing their own personal assistants; to train disabled people to undertake consumer audit in local authorities and other services; to reach out to disabled people, particularly young people and those who are most disadvantaged; to help them take control of their lives; and to provide personal development courses and a mentoring service. It also has an extensive database of information produced in accessible formats. The SCIL is a member of the British Organisation of Disabled People and actively campaigns on issues of concern to disabled people. The organization has been active in campaigning for comprehensive disability discrimination legislation and is currently involved in a campaign against disabled people being charged for essential community care services. The SCIL is also involved in research, for instance that undertaken by the National Centre for Independent Living, which aims to identify disabled people's support needs.

It is clear from this account that the services offered by this and other CILs differ from those of statutory and traditional voluntary services by taking a broader view of the meaning of disability and acting upon it. The emphasis is not just on health and social care, although this is viewed as very important, but on broader issues such as employment, education, leisure and all aspects of independent living. The SCIL, and many other CILs, are overtly political and are actively involved in campaigning and research to better the lives of disabled people.

From their research Barnes & Mercer (2006) found user-controlled organizations, including CILs, to be more accountable to disabled people than statutory and voluntary organizations, and more responsive to their needs both in terms of what is offered and how it is offered. User-controlled organizations are more likely to enhance user choice and control and are more aware and sensitive to the impact of physical and social barriers. Barnes & Mercer (2006:135) state that 'Although lacking the resources to provide a fully comprehensive service, CIL-type services are regarded as substantially more receptive to disabled people's needs'.

You may have noted that some of the work that CILs are engaged in is similar to that of professionals such as physiotherapists and occupational therapists. For instance, CILS are involved in aids and equipment, counselling, advocacy and research.

Local authorities have been reluctant to invest in CILs that struggle with inadequate and insecure funding (Hasler 2006). Compared with statutory services their funding is very low making it difficult for them to fulfil all of their objectives and to be competitive (Barnes & Mercer 2006). Furthermore, if self-funding is increased, by providing disability equality training for example, local authorities are liable to cut the financial contribution they make. User-controlled organizations are also relatively few in number and there is no formal system of referral from other organizations. Barnes & Mercer (2006) found 84 user-controlled organizations in their research, of which 22 were CILs. They state (2006:121):

> Most disabled people across Britain remain reliant upon a bewildering array of services delivered by a variety of statutory and voluntary agencies generally, but not exclusively, controlled and run by non-disabled professionals and dominated by a culture of 'social care' rather than social right.

Although a good collaborative relationship can be developed between statutory services and CILs, the reliance of CILs on statutory funding can cause problems. Local authorities may, for example, insist that CILs define the people they work with in terms of impairment that is anathema to those working within a social model philosophy. Local authorities may also monitor performance in terms of quantitative criteria that may not be appropriate for the type of work CILs are engaged in – a problem which therapists working in certain fields may also experience. It has also been argued that professionals working within statutory services, such as social workers, 'colonize' the ideas and initiatives of disabled people, modifying them and taking them over as their own. Centres for Independent Living may, for example, provide statutory and voluntary services with knowledge about disabled people employing personal assistants, which they then use to undercut CILs when competing for contracts (Barnes & Mercer 2006). Ian Loynes, the coordinator of SCIL, states 'There are many traditional charities circling like vultures and therefore we all have to work hard to stop our revolution from dying' (SCIL 2006:15).

Political campaigning, particularly if it involves direct action, can also be problematic for organizations that are dependent on statutory bodies for some of their funding. Once their ideas and policies are incorporated into the mainstream political agenda their radical edge may be lost (Barnes & Mercer 2006). Some user-led groups, for example Disability Action North East, have avoided statutory funding in order to be autonomous, although this leaves them vulnerable – indeed this particular organization has recently been disbanded for financial reasons.

Equally as important as the many practical services CILs provide is the challenge they pose to traditional services. Drake (1996:190) states that CILs '… have proved a cogent and powerful alternative to the traditional gamut of projects like day centres and social clubs', and Oliver & Zarb (1997:206) believe that CILs represent '… an explicit critique of prevailing social structures and the position of disabled people within them'. Centres for Independent Living also show that disabled people, rather than being passive victims, are capable of running their own affairs. As Finkelstein (1991:34) states:

> The fact that the centres and the services they provide have been devised and delivered by disabled people … presents a positive and rigorous public image contradicting the general depiction of disabled people as a burden on the state and an appropriate focus for the attention of charity.

Centres for Independent Living have arisen from the personal and political struggles of disabled people and have engaged statutory authorities in a social model approach. They have also blurred the distinction between users and providers (Priestley 1999). Barnes (1991:223) states that CILs:

> represent a unique attempt to achieve self-empowerment as well as being a form of direct action aimed at creating new solutions to problems defined by disabled people themselves.

CHANGING THERAPY PRACTICE

Activity 7.6

HOW CAN THERAPY PRACTICE CHANGE

Without compromising any of your present skills, consider some of the ways in which your practice could change to capture the spirit and practice of CILs.

The issue of change within the physiotherapy and occupational therapy professions takes us back to our earlier discussion of power. As you saw in Chapter 5, disabled people value the skills and expertise that therapists have to offer but they need to be in an equal partnership where their knowledge, skills and experience are equally valid and where disability is viewed as a social and political phenomenon. The philosophy and practice of CILs show how different services become when disabled people take control and when the complexities of disability are fully acknowledged. Such a change of orientation may not be easy for therapists. As Pound (2004:37) states, 'relocating the source of disablement as within the social and medical environment is a stern challenge to a therapist's hard won status and accoutrements of power'.

It is not at all easy for individual therapists to change practice in substantial ways, as change depends on the ability to exercise power as well as the historical and social context wherein the therapy is placed. As Welshman (2006:18) states, 'There is a long time lag between ideas and implementation'. To give an example, the National Council for Civil Liberties exposed exploitation of people with learning difficulties within institutions in their book *Outside the Law* in 1951 but, as we have seen, the numbers of people in mental deficiency hospitals rose well into the 1970s. However, as Walmsley (2006b:55), talking of these institutions, states, 'Although it is important to stress that ideas alone did not drive change, they did create mental frameworks within which change was conceptualised'.

As noted in earlier chapters, there is often a mismatch between the ideas and objectives of professionals and those of disabled people that has led many disabled people to regard professionals with suspicion. Walmsley (2006b:48) states, for instance, that 'disability activists have rejected the idea that care is what they need as opposed to receiving assistance to lead the types of lives they choose as active and equal citizens'. Pound (2004:37), a disabled speech and language therapist, reflects that 'People who came for therapy and celebrated their difference were regarded as "poorly adjusted" and "lacking in insight".' She goes on to state that (2004:36):

> Role models within rehabilitation and the media were those who worked hard and battled to overcome the odds, not those who struggled with anger, challenged the power of medicine and demonstrated pride and confidence in self-management techniques.

Kagan & Duchan (2004) gathered the views of people with aphasia to discover what made speech and language therapy work for them. As well as wanting the therapy to improve their language skills, they were also concerned that it should impact on their independence, relationships, self-esteem, feelings of optimism and hope for the future, control of life and the ability to help others. Kagan & Duchan (2004:170) state that:

> Current approaches to consumer involvement in aphasia service provision tend to be confined to having customers evaluate the quality of the service. Our customers focused more on life participation topics, such as whether the services resulted in people getting out and about more, having satisfying relationships and being more independent … Our customers treated communication in social terms focusing on life participation dimensions.

Lyon (2004:80) believes that:

> aphasia treatments need to be more life-orientated and life altering to endure … they need to 'fit' with the life schemes and agendas of those affected. They need ultimately to make those who receive them feel better about themselves, their lives, their connections with others. Certainly addressing disruptive communication is essential … but we must place our first priority in what in life is most desired.

Although these writers are talking about people with aphasia, we believe that their ideas are equally applicable to disabled people with other impairments as well as to other therapists. The following list of ideas for good practice with disabled clients, modified from Pound (2004:40–45), provides a starting point for therapists who wish to practise more inclusively and holistically:

- Acknowledge the full impact of the context and culture on the content of therapy and how clients perceive it.
- Acknowledge how narratives, for instance those which concentrate on cure, infuse therapy.
- Acknowledge the role of power and status in therapy.

- Engage clients in activities over and above their conventional role within therapy, for instance as trainers.
- Exploit fun and creativity.
- Give information and locate wide sources of help, making sure it is fully accessible.
- Advocate for clients and help them to advocate for themselves.
- Stimulate group work where, for instance, clients may gain support from each other and have the opportunity to tell their stories and listen to those of others. As Pound (2004:45) states:

> Create the conditions that allow for more than a 'patient–therapist' relationship. Boundaries are important but enabling someone to feel like a person as opposed to a patient and modelling person-to-person (not therapist-to-patient) interaction is a powerful tool for supporting re-engagement with non-patient life and roles.

- Be willing and confident in spending time with others in the rehabilitation process.
- Frequently acknowledge the client's expertise and do not overpower clients with your own expertise.
- Value the impact of authentic and responsive listening.
- Be prepared to change your view in response to the views of service users.

CONCLUSION

This chapter has examined the meaning of 'profession' and the role of professionals in the lives of disabled people. Disabled people want and expect the best medical care available to them, if and when it is necessary, but they also expect to be treated as equals and as full participative citizens in control of their own lives. The disabled people's movement has always welcomed non-disabled people as allies, supporters and colleagues but is no longer prepared to accept services which do not involve them and which do not meet their needs and rights. This has led Penn (2004:85) to believe that 'No effective therapist can be neutral politically'. This leaves therapists with a dilemma and a choice which are captured in the words of Whalley Hammell (2006:197–198), an occupational therapist, in her book on disability and rehabilitation:

> … an individualised, function-obsessed, approach to rehabilitation is an inadequate response to the circumstances that confront disabled people in their everyday lives. In conjunction with attention to the personal impact of impairment … rehabilitation

practitioners need to focus on the social impact of disability: challenging socially constructed 'norms', contesting marginalisation and exploitation, striving for equality of opportunity and for respect for human rights ... a sole focus on impairment fails to address the reality of disability.

Such a change would involve a redefinition of the role of physiotherapists and occupational therapists, both in practice and philosophy, at all levels of the profession and medical infrastructure. Every therapist can, however, enact change in their practice straight away while those who hold power in policy making and education could, with energy and political will, and in close collaboration with disabled people, pioneer a service which disabled people would embrace.

Chapter 8

What is empowerment?

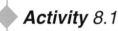

Activity 8.1

WHAT IS EMPOWERMENT?

What does the term 'empowerment' mean to you personally? What does it mean in therapy practice?

We have posed this question at the beginning of the chapter in order for you to set down a marker of your present understanding. This will serve as a starting point for considering the issues discussed below. We are confident that you will have an existing view, as the term *empowerment* has become so ubiquitous across all areas of health and social care. For instance, empowerment, according to the Department of Health (1991), is the driving force within contemporary UK health and social services. The concept of empowerment is associated with other concepts such as choice, involvement, participation and partnership. It is a contested and complex concept that reaches into day-to-day living and the power relations of which we are all a part.

Three quotations set the scene for this discussion, the first two being definitions of empowerment.

In a book about health promotion, empowerment is defined as follows:

> In essence, empowerment is a process that provides the means for individuals or groups to develop the capacity of choice (Labonte 2004) and become more involved in, able to take control of and make decisions about personal or community health and well-being.
>
> (Scriven 2005:7)

There may seem little that is controversial in this statement. Control and choice within decision making that shapes lives would seem an unquestionable aspiration for individuals and groups.

The second definition is from a dictionary of physiotherapy (Porter 2005:107):

> Empowerment: A process of facilitating people in gaining greater control over their lives, life choices and the social and personal challenges they face. Though empowerment can be facilitated, it is changes experienced by those who gain a sense of control that are crucial to empowerment. In this sense empowerment cannot be 'given', but must be 'taken'.

Comparing the two definitions, the common orientation towards choice and control is clear. In the first definition, however, empowerment is *provided*, presumably by service providers, while in the second it is *taken* by service users.

Contrast these definitions with the following quotation from a disabled activist (Gibbs 2004:149):

> Words like 'empower' and 'enable' (even 're-able', which has entered the modernisation programme like a mystery virus) are used in the sense of something that can be prescribed. This usage must be flatly refuted: from the moment that someone presumes to prescribe and manage another's 'empowerment' they prevent it; from the moment they ask 'how can I empower this person?' they begin to do the opposite.

Gibbs complicates matters further. As we shall see below, what is meant to empower can actually have the opposite effect of being disempowering. 'The opposite' is key for reflection here. The notion of empowerment has meaning as against disempowerment. Similarly to be powerful has meaning in apposition to being powerless. This reaches into the meaning of disability itself. To disable, according to the Concise Oxford Dictionary, is 'to deprive of power' – to disempower. So we will begin with experiences of disempowerment before moving on to empowerment and the possible implications for therapy practice. We conclude by re-examining the concept of empowerment as a driving force of policy and practice in therapy.

WHAT DISEMPOWERS?

Barnes & Bowl define empowerment in terms of broad-ranging transformations in people's lives. Their list includes (2001:25):

- personal growth and development
- gaining greater control over life choices
- resistance to and subversion of dominant discourses and practices
- a means of achieving structural change: reducing inequalities
- a process of developing and valuing different knowledges – linking knowledge and action – praxis.

Looking at this list, we find it difficult to relate to day-to-day experiences, and expect that you may feel similarly. Is it possible to be specific, for instance, about 'gaining greater control over life choices' or 'achieving structural change: reducing inequalities'? The lack of clear meaning has underpinned critiques of the overuse of the term as jargon or buzzword, and its use in justifying questionable practices.

For many disabled people the search for empowerment begins with, and is generated by, the experience of disempowerment. Civil and human rights, as history shows, were pushed onto the political agenda by those whose rights were denied, transgressed and infringed. Likewise, for disabled people, empowerment means challenging their disempowerment however it is manifest – through poverty, segregation, institutionalization, institutionalized abuse and discrimination and restrictions on life choices. So let us explore experiences of disempowerment, as it is in relation to this that empowerment has meaning.

◆ *Activity* *8.2*

WHAT DISEMPOWERS YOU?

Give one example of a personal experience in which you felt disempowered. In what ways was it disempowering and what do you think made it disempowering?

In terms of Barnes & Bowl's (2001) definition above, this would be an experience that:

- restricted personal growth and development
- reduced control over life choices
- was determined by dominant discourses and practices
- reinforced the status quo of inequalities
- restricted thinking and different possibilities for action.

In discussions with students, mostly non-disabled health professionals, a number of themes consistently arise, including the following:

- Recurrent disempowering experiences as service users. Women's experiences during pregnancy and giving birth are the most often cited examples of personal disempowerment. Experiences with the care of elderly relatives is another common theme.

- Discussions have also centred around experiences which may be thought of as disempowering but are not necessarily so. Some students, for instance, talk about recurrent derogatory remarks from teachers and how they fuelled their determination to succeed and achieve professional status.

◆ *Activity 8.3*

A PERSONAL EPIPHANY

Personal epiphanies are moments and experiences in a person's life that change or leave marks on the individual. Maureen Gillman wrote the following story. As you read, write down your thoughts about its implications for understanding disempowerment.

When I was ten years old, I went with my mother to see a consultant ophthalmologist at a local hospital. After examination he told my mother, in my presence, that my sight was very poor and likely to deteriorate further. His advice to my mother was that I would never amount to much and should be guided away from employment in which I would need to read and write. He thought some kind of practical work with my hands would be a suitable direction for me. My mother was incensed by this advice and, with a rather rude word to the consultant, we left. I can remember her indignation and her subsequent determination to refute this predicted future for me and I recall a growing determination, on my part, to prove him wrong. The consultant's predictions about my sight proved to be accurate and I am now registered blind. However, his prophecy about my abilities and subsequent employment have not materialized. I stayed in mainstream education and eventually trained to be a social worker. Since then I have obtained a PhD and I am employed as a Principal lecturer at a University.

(French et al 2001:222–223)

In this story the dichotomy between empowerment and disempowerment breaks down. Looking from the professional's viewpoint, his purpose could be seen as facilitating empowerment, though he was unlikely to have used the term then. He provided facts based on his supposed expertise so Maureen and her family could be realistic in their expectations and life choices. From an outsider viewpoint, the experience could be seen as disempowering, limiting choice, possibilities and opportunities. From the viewpoint of Maureen and her family, the experience was empowering in the sense that it set them on a path of self-empowerment in opposition to the consultant's presumptions.

The notion of empowerment, then, is highly complex and debatable. Returning to the quotation from Gibbs (2004) above, not only can the provision of empowerment be disempowering, ostensibly disempowering experiences can be empowering. We need to look a little further at the term 'disempowerment' as it clearly does have meaning in disabled people's lives, particularly at what it might mean to be lacking in power.

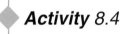

Activity 8.4

WHAT DOES IT MEAN TO BE POWERLESS?

The following draws on an oral history project conducted with over 60 visually impaired people who gave detailed accounts, telling stories of their experiences of education (French & Swain 2006). As you read, write down your thoughts on people's experiences of lacking power.

Ray, as other participants, described the heavy regimentation of bedtimes:

Bedtime was very regimented to the extent that you fell into categories so you had 'six o'clockers', 'half past sixers', 'seven o'clockers' and when you got to about 13, the latest you could go was nine o'clock.

(p. 386)

Peter described a similar regimented regime in a school run by nuns:

You weren't allowed to talk at meal times unless they said we could. You had to account for every single thing at ... [the school], you had to be in a given place, at a given time at all times. There was no choice about anything at all, You had to eat what you were given, you weren't allowed to leave food. A lot of people were sick there because they were made to eat things that didn't agree with them.

(p. 386)

Many factors were thought to play a part, including religion. Mary recalled:

... you really had religion rammed down your throat. Jane (Mary's twin sister) was sent outside the door because she didn't understand what 'secure from all our fears' meant in 'Lord keep us safe this night'. She thought it was 'sick your' instead of 'secure', but at seven you don't understand these words.

(p. 387)

This regimentation reverberated through these young people's lives and relationships, including their relationships with other pupils. Returning to Mary's story she told us:

Jane and I had each other but the time we were put on silence I wasn't even allowed to speak to her. I think Jane's depression started from those days, she'd vomit for no apparent reason.

(p. 387)

Jane takes up the story:

The adults resented the relationship I had with Mary, they didn't like us being affectionate. Even if one of us was ill they wouldn't let us comfort each other. I can remember when I first started the depression I was really ill and Mary was cuddling me and this teacher came up and said 'Let go of each other, go up to the surgery Jane.' It was awful. We weren't allowed to see each other if we were in sick bay. We hated not being together.

(p. 387)

The lack of emotional involvement, with some rare exceptions, characterized relationships between young children and the staff acting 'in loco parentis'. Rob explained:

It was a pretty tough regime, Dickensian I think would be the word. There was a matron who wore a long white overall with a flowing white hat ... . She was extremely strict religiously and I couldn't stand her.

(p. 387)

Sometimes specific individuals were named, though Mary's account still sets the focus on the institution:

There was one girl, June her name was, and for whatever reason she would wet herself occasionally, and Miss H used to really lay into June. When you're a child you accept it because you think it's normal, you think it's the way people treat other people, you don't realise that there is anything wrong with it, you accept it as a normal way for adults to behave. I can see from that angle how abused people can become abusers because they think it's the normal way to carry on.

(p. 387)

Mary also recalled the denial of privacy, another common abusive experience in these participants' stories:

We could have our own radio but I had mine taken away from me for a week because I played it somewhere where I shouldn't have done. It was so stupid, it really was. Another rule was that we weren't allowed to go upstairs into the dormitory during the day. When I got to a certain age, and was allowed to wash my own hair, I would always ask permission to wash my hair on a Wednesday evening so I could listen to a certain programme that was on. It was as silly as that. There was nowhere private, you had no privacy whatsoever, privacy was nil.

(p. 387)

Even letters to parents were censored, though perhaps it is not surprising in such total institutions, where abuse is ingrained into everyday experience. Carol's letters home were read and censored and her personal possessions checked:

> I hated having things like drawer check. I don't see why you can't keep your things in a mess in your drawer. In those days you didn't you just did what they said and you were in big trouble if you didn't. You had loss of privileges which meant you couldn't go out so it was a big drawback if you didn't do as you were told.
>
> (p. 388)

In Peter's school, run by Catholic nuns, the scrutiny of every aspect of day-to-day life seemed to know no bounds:

> They were very, very strict about modesty and that sort of thing. For instance as soon as you stood up from the bath you were expected to wrap a towel round your waist so that you couldn't look at yourself while you were drying yourself. Even the totally blind kids had to do all this. There were also very strict routines about cleanliness and so on. Not in the sense of having baths every day, we only had a bath once a week and we only changed our socks and underwear once a week, but they were obsessed with our hair being clean. We used to have our hair fine combed with one of those metal combs twice a term and they used to use this horrible, green liquid stuff. The nuns were quite vicious, I can remember my scalp being quite badly scraped and scratched by those combs. With regard to the underwear they would come round every Saturday to collect your dirty laundry and they would inspect your underpants and if there were any 'skid marks' you were made to go off and wash them under the supervision of one of the nuns, even quite small boys had to do that. It was really horrible especially for the blind kids because they didn't always realise.
>
> (p. 388)

Young (1990) defines powerlessness as a lack of decision-making power, a lack of capacity to enact choices and a marginal status through disrespectful treatment. Though these disabled people were not specifically asked to talk about powerlessness, they speak with eloquence about lacking power from experiences.

In theory there are two related directions in thinking about lacking power. The first focuses on the person: the person is rendered powerless. A theoretical basis for this is in the work of Seligman (1975). His theory of learned helplessness basically argues that people who are repeatedly subjected to experiences where they have no control are rendered powerless. It is a theory of the psychological price of powerlessness in which oppression becomes internalized. There are three debilitating effects. The first is a lack of motivation to try to control events. If people have learnt that they have little effect on valued outcomes or undesired events, they will cease to try to solve problems or overcome barriers. Second, the emotional effects typically involve depression, resignation and anxiety. Third, there is also a general disruption to learning that involves people having difficulty in understanding that their behaviour does have consequences. Even when success is experienced, a person will have difficulty learning that what he or she does actually affects outcomes or events (Swain 1989).

The theory of learned helplessness provides only a partial explanation of powerlessness and is questionable. It focuses on 'helplessness' as a condition of the individual. By concentrating on psychological responses the danger is that the victim is blamed – the disabled person is 'helpless'. It might also be explained as psychological survival. If going against the rules leads to punishment, complying may be the most logical thing to do. In institutions, what looks like learned helplessness may be nothing more than a sensible strategy to survive.

The second orientation in understanding powerlessness centres on the power relations that are built into our society. Davey (1999:38) summarizes this as follows:

> Powerlessness has economic, environmental, social, interpersonal, health, emotional and cognitive dimensions. Powerless people live in limiting physical surroundings; they are spatially and socially separated from people and places that decide about their destiny; they are not 'well connected'; they have lower purchasing power as consumers, no purchasing power for entrepreneurial and investment roles …

From this viewpoint then, powerlessness is political rather than just personal. Disabled people are rendered powerless through segregation, institutionalization, isolation, inferior education, poverty, lack of information, environmental and attitudinal barriers – restrictions on opportunities and choices. The above extracts from the history project clearly speak to the politics of powerlessness. The participants are speaking from experiences of institutionalization, itself an expression of the lack of opportunities, resources and support. They are speaking too from experiences of powerlessness within residential care.

Powerlessness and the process of disempowerment are both personal and political, though they are intertwined. One possible understanding of the inter-relationship is a re-interpretation of the causes of learned helplessness. Thus Swain (1989:116) states:

> What may seem to be enduring, debilitating characteristics of the people – such as apathy, fatalism, depression and pessimism – are

actually 'the straightforward manifestation of the dynamics arising from lack of power'.

WHAT EMPOWERS?

We turn, then, to address directly the question set by the title of this chapter, what is empowerment, building on our discussions of disempowerment and powerlessness. As we have seen disabled people can be rendered powerless by recurrent processes, for example institutionalization, and they can need time, support and resources to build up sufficient confidence to participate fully. Thus we concentrate, as will become clearer, on processes of empowerment, so the question becomes: what is empowering?

Looking towards the literature, it seems that the term 'empowerment' has many meanings and, as Gomm suggests, has become something of a buzzword, used differently in different contexts by different people towards their own ends. He writes (1993:6):

> What can we do with a term which on the right of politics can mean privatising public services, and on the far left can mean abolishing private services; which can mean all things to all men, and something different again to some women?

Whatever the specific definition, the term 'empowerment' is widespread. It pervades academic and professional literature, policy statements emanating from organizations of disabled people as well as large-scale charity organizations for disabled people and professional organizations. For instance, the Prime Minister's Strategy Unit (2005:70) states:

> Disabled people stress that, just because someone might need assistance to go about their daily life, this does not mean they have to be 'dependent'. Independence comes from having choice and being empowered regarding the assistance needed. Without this choice and empowerment, disabled people are unable to fulfil their roles and responsibilities as citizens.

This quotation rightly complicates matters even further, as empowerment is associated with other complex and contested ideas, for instance independence and citizenship. It is clear from our exploration of notions of disempowerment that empowerment cannot be translated into a clear set of agreed practices, as a 'cookbook' or recipe that renders disabled people empowered. What empowers is, rather, addressed through a set of principles underlying practice. Principles are ideals towards which therapy practice is directed and against which practice is reflected upon (Swain et al 2004a). Here we shall suggest just four:

1. Empowerment is a process that promotes people's prediction and control over decision making that shapes their lives

Defining empowerment, Thompson (1998:211) is succinct:

> We can identify its core element as a process of helping people gain greater control over their lives and the sociopolitical and existential challenges they face.

Thus empowerment is viewed as a continuing process of change rather than a product that is or is not achieved. This clearly applies to other notions in current disability policy such as independence and inclusion. They are processes that are worked towards.

As suggested by Thompson (1998), control is central to empowerment. Control can be through choices, but choices can be limited by what is on offer – and those decisions can be elsewhere, in the hands of powerful people. Davey (1999:39) takes a far-reaching view of control:

> To me it means a situation in which disadvantaged groups or individuals begin to define purposes for themselves and then plan, design, implement and monitor a change process.

2. Empowerment is the questioning of power relations, organizational structures and dominant ways of understanding that limit people's life choices and control (i.e. that disempower)

Empowerment in this sense is a challenge to professionals and the power structures of the provision of services. Hugman (1991:38) provides a detailed analysis and states:

> If power is not an isolated element of social life, but one which interweaves occupational and organisational structures with the actions of professionals, individually and collectively, then it must be examined in terms of the contexts within which the caring professions are structured and operate.

Empowerment from this viewpoint is a process of challenging and changing institutional and organizational structures, the work of professionals, rather than changing individual service users. It also involves challenging dominant understandings, particularly the medical model, with its emphasis on the 'personal tragedy' of disability. The aim is that the system becomes more empowering or less disempowering.

3. Empowerment is political as well as personal in promoting people's struggles against 'man-made' sufferings and the removal of barriers to equal opportunities and full participatory citizenship

As disempowerment is both personal and political, empowerment is the mirror image. Davey (1999:37), amongst others, looks towards a broader framework:

> Empowerment must address all their [disabled people's] problems together if it is to be meaningful. Poverty, poor housing and the nature of the social security system put a strain on relationships and lead to widespread demoralisation. Depending on the circumstances of individuals they can lead to physical and mental ill health, criminality, addiction and the persecution of individual or collective scapegoats: racism, sexism, picking on individuals.

Problems are seen as having social origins: poverty, bad housing, unremitting child care and care of old people without adequate support. Growth and change are seen as being fostered in non-hierarchical and co-operative relationships in which differences are accepted and, indeed, celebrated. Such relationships provide a safe and supportive space for people to explore and express their feelings and thoughts and to come to their own understandings of the oppression faced through the inequalities and hierarchies in society. This empowers people, in principle at least, to contribute to the transforming of hierarchical relationships and thus the changing of society. Standing (1999), a physiotherapist working with people with learning difficulties, writes of the possibilities for empowerment through working in partnership with clients. She states (1999:256):

> Empowerment is likely to be achieved in situations and within programmes where professionals are not the key actors. The cognitive, motivational and personality changes experienced by those who gain a sense of control are the essence of empowerment.

Personal and political empowerment are not separate processes but totally intertwined: each generates the other.

4. Empowerment is taken by those who are powerless rather than given by those who have power

Empowerment is not a gift from those who have power to those who have been rendered powerless. Priestley (1999:165) states that:

> The message from the disabled people's movement is that empowerment is not something that can be 'done to' disabled

people by others. Rather it is something that they must do for themselves through self-organisation, collective self-advocacy, direct action and self-managed personal support.

Empowerment, then, is political in terms of both the problems addressed and the solutions or possibilities for change. In the light of these principles, we can now look at specific possibilities or strategies for empowerment. We turn first to therapeutic encounters. Reynolds (2004c:125) provides a succinct overview:

> Communications that support clients' decision-making and control are central to empowerment. The 'building blocks' of good communication … such as active listening, providing information and inviting clients to contribute to the therapeutic encounter through open questions, all enhance clients' participation in decision-making and their ability to control outcomes.

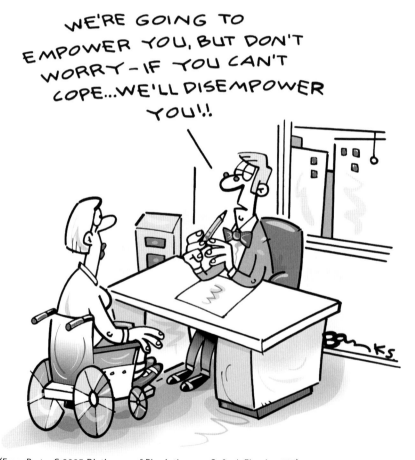

(From Porter S 2005 Dictionary of Physiotherapy, Oxford, Elsevier, 107)

There are numerous examples of strategies and frameworks for developing empowering practice (for example, Ashton & Rodgers 2005). The following is a summary of the common 'building blocks':

- The development of an equal professional–client relationship in which both bring their expertise to the therapeutic encounter.
- The beliefs, values, feelings and opinions of the disabled person are considered important and actively sought.
- The disabled person should be encouraged to influence the content of meetings, initially by being asked to identify specific issues that impact on their self-care.
- Disabled people should generate the solutions to the issues they identify to ensure that interventions fit into the context of their lifestyles, values and support systems.

This orientation towards empowerment comes largely from professionals. It concentrates on personal empowerment, although it does challenge the therapeutic process. As Beresford (2006:596) observes:

> Professional approaches to empowerment have been particularly concerned with *personal* empowerment. Personal empowerment is concerned with people being able to develop new and different understandings of themselves and their world, so they are better equipped to respond to opportunities to take power.

Nevertheless, notions of empowerment have been developed in professional practice in many different ways. There is certainly no 'royal road' for therapists to follow in either empowering themselves or supporting the empowerment of others. One route explored by Ghaye & Lillyman is reflective conversation. They state (2000:64):

> Reflective conversations which are empowering enable us to name, define and construct our own 'realities', to gain a greater sense of control over our professional lives and to develop a more authentic self.

In their framework, reflective conversation is at the heart of the process of reflecting on practice. Reflective conversation between colleagues can be empowering for therapists. According to Ghaye & Lillyman (2000) the prime focus is on caring values, reflecting on your intentions in the therapy process – the ends you have in mind and the means for achieving them. There seem to be two associations with empowerment for clients:

1. Reflective conversations prioritize the meaning and value of the clients' viewpoint – what they bring to therapy, the meaning of therapy for clients and their evaluation of therapy in relation to their lives.

2. Critical reflection is creative in terms of support for clients in control over decision making within the therapy process.

Another context that can be thought to offer more opportunities for empowerment than one-to-one therapeutic encounters is group work. Group situations can provide contexts for supporting and affirming positive identity and self-worth. The group context can broaden the possibilities for empowerment, moving from the personal towards the political, in moving from the individual towards the collective. Reynolds (2004d:139) provides the following list of possible empowering experiences within group contexts in which this broadening of possibilities is evident:

- Empathy, acceptance and validation.
- Expert advice and information.
- Emotional and practical support.
- Challenge and a stimulus for change.
- Opportunities to take on valued roles.
- Social facilitation effects and role modelling.
- Developing social skills and insights.
- Transcendence – moving beyond self.
- Consciousness raising and political activism.

CONNECT, an organization which works with people with aphasia to provide appropriate services as they define them, is an example of this approach. Sally Byng, the chief executive, states (Swain et al 2003:96):

> It feels like people with aphasia are taking ownership of this place ... I really believe that what we have done is create the condition for them to do what they want.

Reynolds (2004d) also takes us towards collective empowerment and political activism, which has found its most far-reaching expression through the growth of the disabled people's movement. Charlton (2000:117) goes as far as to suggest that 'The only way to empowerment is through the conscious activity of people themselves. This is one lesson that all oppressed groups have had to learn'.

It is widely recognized by disabled people that the growth of the disabled people's movement reflects and engenders the individual and collective empowerment of disabled people (Campbell & Oliver 1996). Part of this process is consciousness raising towards an altered understanding of self and others. This involves a re-interpretation of experiences and identity. The collective sharing of experiences affirms commonalities and re-interprets the problem away from the supposedly tragic individual, to the treatment of people with impairments in a disabling society. In this way, the social model of disability, in direct contrast to individual, medical and tragedy models, is seen by disabled people as the model of empowerment. As you saw in Chapter 2, the social model sees disability not as a personal tragedy nor an individual problem, but as a societal issue; the consequences of the barriers – structural, environmental and attitudinal – which society imposes upon people with impairments. The empowerment comes, then, from disabled people themselves rather than being a gift from those in power.

Crow (1996:206–207), in a chapter reflecting critically on the social model, makes the following statement that does not use the term empowerment but clearly affirms the role of the social model in empowering disabled people:

> For years now this social model of disability has enabled me to confront, survive and even surmount countless situations of exclusion and discrimination. It has been my mainstay, as it has been for the wider disabled people's movement. It has enabled a vision of ourselves free from the constraints of disability (oppression) and provided a direction for our commitment to social change. It has played a central role in promoting disabled people's individual self-worth, collective identity and political organisation. I don't think it is an exaggeration to say that the social model has saved lives.

Thus the collective self-empowerment by disabled people addresses issues of both personal and political change.

THERAPY AND EMPOWERMENT

To conclude this chapter we turn to critical reflection on the specific role of the therapist in facilitating empowerment. First let us look at the possible barriers faced by therapists in adopting a positive role.

Activity 8.5

WHAT ARE THE BARRIERS FACED BY THERAPISTS?

List the barriers that you face or might face in facilitating the empowerment of service users through therapy practice. It may help if you look back to the principles and possible strategies covered in the previous section of this chapter.

There are numerous barriers you might have identified. Looking from the viewpoint of a disabled activist, Davis (1999:20) captures the barriers to self-empowerment as follows:

> Throughout the years of disabled people's self-organisation and collective struggle, what has been most fundamentally amiss boils down to two main issues. First, a limpet-like attachment by the disability establishment to a 'medical model' view of disability; second, the disproportionate distribution of power and influence between those who control disability policy and disabled people themselves.

The barriers you might have identified could be a mirror image of these. Certainly the dominance of the medical model underpins individual expectations and attitudes, the cultural context of therapy practice and the training received by therapists. Much of the practice of occupational therapists and physiotherapists has been within the framework of the medical model. Empowerment within this context means getting the individual to be able to do as much for him- or herself as possible, and often this will be the criterion for discharge or judging the success of treatment. Empowerment, within a medical framework, is judged on whether the patient can do things for him- or herself, whether he or she can dress, cook, wash and so on. This notion of empowerment does not sit comfortably with empowerment as defined through the four principles outlined above or with the philosophy of the disabled people's movement or the social model of disability.

It has been argued by some that professionals may lack the power to change services and practices (Warren 1999). Professionals typically operate within hierarchical, top–down management systems and institutional change can be slow and difficult to influence at least from the lower rungs of the ladder.

There is an argument too that the notion of empowerment begs complex questions. Is it equally applicable across all cultures, for instance with people from ethnic minority communities? Can it be applied to the lives of all disabled people? Clegg suggests that empowerment is unobtainable for most people with learning difficulties. She states:

> Empowerment imposes the liberal value of autonomy onto intellectually disabled people inappropriately: unattainable for most, autonomy erases mutuality and relationships from their lives. (2006:13)

Again, then, we need to return to the principles outlined above. Empowerment is an ideal. There are barriers from both sides – for therapists and service users. It depends crucially on the breaking down of the unequal power relations, and working together in partnership.

Activity 8.6

THE POSSIBLE IMPLICATIONS OF EMPOWERMENT FOR THERAPY PRACTICE

In the final activity for this chapter we end on a positive note. Give one example of therapy practice, from your experience, which you feel was empowering for a service user. In what ways was it empowering and what do you think made it empowering?

Perhaps not surprisingly, given the complexities we have discussed, there is little empirical insight into how empowerment is facilitated in practice (Scriven 2005). Your own experiences, if critically reflected on, are the best foundation for good practice, through working with others (service users and service providers). This brings us to the topic of partnership which we shall discuss in the next chapter.

Chapter 9

What is partnership?

AFFILIATION, COLLABORATION, PARTICIPATION, ALLIANCE?

The title of this chapter may seem to set a simple, or simplistic, question. It addresses the meaning of what is an everyday term. Most, if not all, of us are or have been in relationships of one kind or another that can be deemed partnerships: 'family' relationships, with a partner of the opposite or same sex, working partnerships with colleagues, in our case a writing partnership, business partnerships, political partnerships and so on. As a starting point for exploring issues generated by this question, let us begin with this general everyday usage of the term.

Activity 9.1

THE QUALITIES OF PARTNERSHIPS

Think of a partnership that you are presently involved in, or have been involved in, and list the qualities of this relationship. What makes it an effective partnership?

We have a working, writing partnership that is effective for us both. Some of the qualities of our partnership may correspond to those you listed, though we are certainly not suggesting that ours is a definitive list:

- It has endured. We have written together for over 15 years.
- It is grounded in a strong personal relationship of mutual respect and shared values.
- It is open and continually negotiated and renegotiated.
- We both value the relationship.
- It is open to different ways of working. Co-authoring is a complex process that can be conducted in numerous ways. We have kept these open.
- As partners we deal together with the publishing system.
- We can challenge each other and strengthen our work through sharing our views.
- We support each other in many different ways.

Our particular focus in this chapter is, of course, the notion of partnership in the provision of services for disabled people. As we saw above, whatever it means in policy or practice, it is a term that has a positive connotation in everyday usage and it is a term that can be applied to quite different relationships.

In recent policy developments, 'partnership' has been a dominant concept signifying the attainment of greater equality in professional–client relations generally. At a policy level, partnership and collaborative working are considered to be desirable. Governments of all persuasions have placed emphasis on the need for different agencies to work together to provide more 'seamless' service provision by moving towards more integrated health and social care provision (Department of Health 2000, Department of Health & Department of the Environment 1992).

As we saw with the term empowerment, partnership in terms of policy, practice and provision has become a buzzword, widely accepted as an imperative in the development of services for disabled people and other service users. But acceptance can deflect critical reflection as Mullender & Ward (1991:35) point out in relation to empowerment:

> Because it creates a vogue image and an aura of moral superiority, it offers protection against criticism. Yet the term lacks specificity and is a 'social aerosol' covering up the smell of conflict and conceptual division.

Defining the concept of partnership is difficult because partnership means different things to different groups of people. Looked at broadly, it refers to organizations or individuals working together or acting jointly. Carnwell & Buchanan (2005:6) provide a definition that resonates with everyday usage of the term:

> Shared commitment, where all partners have a right and an 'obligation' to participate and will be affected equally by the benefits and disadvantages arising from the partnership.

To complicate matters, partnership is associated with numerous other terms such as participation and, as we saw in Chapter 8, empowerment. It also encompasses different relationships.

- It refers to the relationship between professionals and between professional organizations. Associated terms include 'inter-agency collaboration', 'joint working' and 'multi-professional practice'. Cohen (2005:2) states:

  > 'Joining-up' is used here in a generic sense to denote the development of a wide range of relationships intended to promote closer and more effective working between services. 'Inter-agency collaboration' is used to refer to a relationship between agencies and services that may involve collaboration in planning, working together on specific issues or projects, or the sharing of posts.

- It refers to the relationship between disabled people or, more particularly, service users and the service system. A key term here is 'service user involvement'. This is again mandated within policy. For instance, one of the Department of Health's six medium-term priorities was that health authorities should:

  > … give greater voice and emphasis to users of NHS services and their carers in their own care, the development and definition of standards set for NHS services locally and the development of NHS policy both locally and nationally.
  >
  > (NHS Executive 1995:9)

- Though much less recognized, the term can be applied to relationships between disabled people, to include partnerships within and between organizations of disabled people. Barnes & Mercer (2006:91–92) state:

  > The gap between disabled people's expectations and their actual involvement in the statutory and voluntary sectors has reinforced claims from disabled people's organizations that the move to a more equal and democratic society demands a bottom-up approach to politics and policy making. Its potential is realised by the emergence of active user-led organisations.

- The term also refers to the more immediate relationship between a professional and a service user. This again can encompass different terms such as 'client-centred practice'. Sumsion (2005:100) defines this as follows:

> In the UK client centred occupational therapy is a partnership between the client and the therapist that empowers the client to engage in functional performance and fulfil their occupational roles in a variety of environments. The client participates actively in negotiating goals that are given priority and are at the centre of assessment, intervention and evaluation.

Providing a more detailed breakdown of the meaning of the term partnership, Reynolds (2004b) suggests that a partnership approach to health care makes the following assumptions:

1. Both professionals and service users are regarded as bringing strengths or resources to the therapeutic process and the therapeutic relationship.

2. Both professionals and service users are part of the team that will openly share information and make decisions about the way forward in therapy.

3. The relationship is respectful and affirmative rather than shaped by dependency, submissiveness or power struggles.

4. The relationship is based on adult strategies of communication, rather than infantilizing, manipulation or stereotyping, with both partners having a respected voice in the interaction.

5. The service user is motivated to share responsibility with the therapist for the therapy process and outcome.

6. The purpose of the partnership is, ostensibly, to promote the service user's self-actualization, development and quality of life rather than pressurizing specifically for better compliance with treatment.

In terms of therapy practice specifically, partnership denotes the inclusion of service users' voices in decision making in the therapy process. The following points are identified by Thompson (1998:213):

1. Identifying problems to be tackled, issues to be addressed, goals to be achieved.
2. Deciding what steps are to be taken and who needs to do what.
3. Undertaking the necessary work through collaboration and consultation.
4. Reviewing progress and agreeing any changes that need to be made to the agreed course of action.
5. Bringing the work to a close if and when necessary.

6. Evaluating the work done, highlighting strengths, weaknesses and lessons to be learned.

◆ *Activity* 9.2

VIEWS OF PARTNERSHIP

The following is an extract from some unpublished research that summarizes some views expressed by visually impaired service users and service providers (Swain et al 2005). As you read, think about the issues raised in relation to partnership.

There was widespread agreement between service users and service providers that the whole system is complex, fragmented and itself creates structural and attitudinal barriers. From the viewpoint of people with visual impairments, the experience of accessing services can be one of frustration from a continuous struggle of searching and being passed on:

> Historically, it has always been the case that the client has to do all the running around and the professionals stay in one place.
>
> (p. 29)

> The attitude of the person on the other end. It's fine when you start, then you get the run around. They don't seem to want to help and they pass you on to someone and then someone else and another section.
>
> (p. 29)

Simply not knowing that help is available seems an important barrier for some people with visual impairments:

> So it is not that people are necessarily frightened to ask for help, it is just that disability label, and also when people do need help they do not necessarily know where to get the help and that is a big problem.
>
> (p. 29)

The need for partnership and collaboration was also clearly and repeatedly emphasised by service providers:

> We really need to be joining together much more but that is about internal communication. I don't know where to go for many things within the council and I work there. How can you expect customers to know? Customers don't see differences between departments and nor should they be expected to when there is a service provider and it is up to us to get together.
>
> (p. 29)

> That's the key to it. It has to be a seamless service where one part links to the other.
>
> (p. 30)

There was some recognition that these particular issues are not confined to the provision of services for people with visual impairments:

> I think perhaps we don't work close enough. We are all in our own little vacuum. We get into that mould because often we are overwhelmed with

> sometimes the amount of work and I'm not looking for excuses. Perhaps it is
> something that we do need to look at but it's not unique to the visual
> impairment world. I think it is perhaps in all disabilities and government
> dealings that they don't work closely together – like the benefits agency.
>
> (p. 30)

The establishment of collaborative joint working is thought to be a priority,
but action strategies for doing so are more problematic. The notion of 'one
stop shop' was alluded to by a number of participants:

> Specialists will be using the same premises but everyone will still have
> their own area of specialization. The main thing is that when you go to
> that office you can ... access everything you need. Like a one stop shop.
>
> (p. 30)

Another suggestion was what might be called a 'one stop supporter':

> If they brought a human interface to the whole system, call it a case
> worker, you are dealing with one person rather than dealing with social
> services, benefit agency ... employment, access issues, specialist
> equipment all the rest of it. You are trying to pull all that together
> yourself. There should be one person, one case worker, who can help you
> to do all of this, to make the whole thing a bit of a goer. But because you
> are having to do it, it makes being disabled bloody tough work and at the
> moment to tell you the truth although the intentions are good, the
> system just doesn't practically work.
>
> (p. 30)

The starting point is clearly deficiencies in the present system of service
provision. The following seem to us to be the general key issues, which
we shall discuss later within this chapter.

Why partnership?

For both service users and service providers the need for a different
relationship lies in the problems experienced within the present system. Partnerships between professionals and service users, for instance,
are predicated on some expectation of an increase in choice for those
receiving services.

The barriers to partnership

Any real choice may be a mirage as choice can be seen as a threat by professionals who act as gatekeepers by continuing to make the decisions
about access to provision. The concept of partnership working cannot be
seen in isolation from the power relations within any partnership. In a partnership, the persons or groups who wield control are the crucial factors

to be recognized. If a shift in power begins to acknowledge that the service user knows best, how does this impact on partnership working?

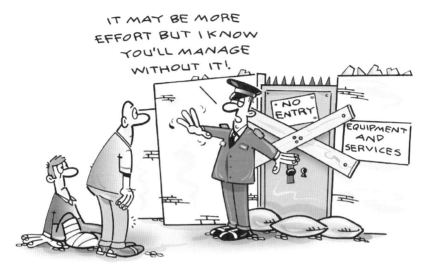

(From Porter S 2005 Dictionary of Physiotherapy, Oxford, Elsevier, 138)

Possibilities for working towards partnership

The key issues here relate to changing organizational structures and establishing effective communication in moving towards a system in which service users can exercise greater control over the services they receive. It can be seen as a continuum, from the involvement and consultation in decision making right through to user control of all processes.

In the remainder of this chapter, then, we shall look first at the reasoning behind this widely accepted notion of partnership. Why partnership? What is the underlying philosophy and how is it manifested in policy and practice? We then turn to the barriers to changing professional organizations and practices and consider what structural, environmental and attitudinal barriers need to be overcome. We conclude by looking towards the possibilities for change and how effective partnerships can be fostered, maintained and evaluated. We shall explore critically the issues from two standpoints: those of service providers and those of service users.

WHY PARTNERSHIP?

The development of user involvement in services for disabled people in the UK can be seen from two stances: that of service providers and that of disabled people. We saw in Chapter 3 that following the election of Margaret Thatcher as Conservative Prime Minister in 1979, there was a shift towards a market ideology in health and social care which was backed by legislation promoting user involvement and partnership. Today the NHS is advocating an empowerment or participation model of helping relationships in which the client's (and carer's) voice is heard, and where health professionals and clients work collaboratively with agreed, shared agendas. User involvement in service planning and evaluation is also, ostensibly, being encouraged. In a review of 12 research programmes, Farrell (2004:2) states:

> Patient involvement increases patient satisfaction. Benefits also include greater confidence, reduction in anxiety, greater under-standing of personal needs, improved trust, better relationships with professionals and positive health effects. Patients feel involved in their care when they are treated as equal partners, listened to and properly informed. Privacy and time for discussion are both required to achieve this.

A number of different models of partnership have been identified, each with its own rationale. Cunningham & Davis (1985) recognize three models of partnership with parents of disabled children, which can be applied on a wider basis. The first is the 'expert model' in which profes-sionals exercise control over intervention and service users are the pas-sive recipients of services. In the 'transplant model' the skills and expertise of professionals as teachers are passed on to parents. It is diffi-cult, however, to see either of these two models of partnership as involv-ing any shifting of power relations. The 'consumer model' allows for a more equal partnership in which the knowledge and rights of service users are recognized. Dale (1996) proposed a fourth model, the 'negotiat-ing model' of partnership. This recognizes that dissent may be a major factor in the relationship between the user and service provider. Dale (1996:14) describes this model as follows:

> a working relationship where the partners use negotiation and joint decision-making and resolve differences of opinion and dis-agreement, in order to reach some kind of shared perspective or jointly agreed decision on issues of mutual concern.

From the viewpoint of service user involvement, Powell & Glendinning (2002) suggest two models. The 'synergy' or 'added value' model focuses on the additional value of combining organizations with their different assets or features. The 'transformation' model focuses on part-ners bringing different capacities to influence the form and direction of the partnerships. The former relates to the consumer model, and the later to the negotiating model.

Coming from the viewpoint of disabled people, the second development was the emergence of well-organized and strengthening user movements, including the disabled people's movement. The agenda of the disabled people's movement goes far beyond the issue of services (however important they may be) to full democratic citizenship and the dismantling of a disabling environment in terms of physical and social barriers (Barton 2004, Campbell & Oliver 1996). Other social movements, such as Survivors Speak Out, Gay Pride, and the self-advocacy movement have similar agendas. Talking of the disabled people's movement, Drake (1996:187) states that:

> it is important to give due weight to the contribution that the disability movement has made in changing the thinking of governments, bringing injustice to light and forcing a radical alteration of the policy agenda.

Carr (2004) also stresses the importance of collectivism in user involvement for disabled people and the ideas and philosophy of the social model of disability that underpin it. The wider consumer culture, and the social forces created by the disabled people's movement, have encouraged this partnership approach.

Standing back from the two viewpoints of the development of service user involvement, there are clear contradictions and controversies that reverberate through the philosophy underpinning partnership. Beresford & Croft note the tension between the ideologies of the government and those of the disabled people's movement. They state (2000:356):

> These two approaches to participation, the consumerist and democratic approaches, do not sit comfortably. One is managerial and instrumental in purpose, without any commitment to the redistribution of power or control, the other liberational with a commitment to empowerment.

BARRIERS TO PARTNERSHIP

There are considerable barriers to working in partnership, whether this is between different groups of professionals or between professionals and service users. The key distinction between the consumerist approach, adhered to by both Conservative and Labour governments since the 1990s, and the democratic/participatory approach taken by the disabled people's movement resounds through the analyses of barriers from different standpoints. Critical reflection in working towards effective partnerships requires the recognition of possibly conflicting perspectives and differing standpoints. We shall look first, then, at the barriers from the viewpoint of service providers.

Activity 9.3

YOUR EXPERIENCES OF BARRIERS

Either from your experience in the clinical setting, or from your general observations as a client, draw up some of the organizational barriers that exist in the NHS which make it difficult for therapists and other staff to establish genuine partnerships with service users. (This activity and the following comments are adapted from Reynolds 2004b:22.)

Numerous organizational barriers to partnership exist within health care. Reynolds (2004b) lists the following:

- The lengthy professional training and, more particularly, socialization of health workers sets up 'social distance' from service users.

- Social constructions of health and health care tend to encourage a focus on pathology, and treatment, rather than considering clients as individuals, i.e. the medical model dominates intervention.

- Resource allocation can result in brief appointments, waiting lists, rationing and withdrawal of certain services, regardless of service users' needs and preferences.

- Some of the values and assumptions driving evidence-based health-care practice distract attention away from the quality of healthcare relationships, particularly as this is a difficult area to measure quantitatively.

The NHS is advocating a partnership approach, not only between health professionals and clients but also among professionals from different disciplines. The goal is to provide a seamless service in which multidisciplinary teams work together to provide maximally effective interventions for clients. Barriers between professionals range from organizational and attitudinal barriers to geographical and financial barriers, which are compounded by the different languages used within heath, education and social care. To bring service users into this equation further serves to add to the complexity of these relationships. The following, then, are some of the possible barriers:

- Rivalry between professionals.

- Waterfield (2004:200) argues that shared skills and knowledge may be problematic for professional groups as they challenge the uniqueness of professionals. She writes, 'There has always been a certain rivalry between physiotherapy and other practitioners such as osteopaths, nurses and occupational therapists.'

- Hierarchical structures have presented important barriers to the effective functioning of multiprofessional teams (French 1999). Different professional agencies may 'fear that someone else may be after their money or taking their job, do not understand or respect the other agency and see them in stereotyped ways' (Heywood 2006:37). Lillywhite (2003) suggests that professionals see their specific skills and areas as unique and are reluctant to allow the boundaries of their role to be challenged by other professionals. As noted in Chapter 7, the development of a specific body of knowledge is thought, by some, to be a defining characteristic of a profession. Distinctive professional allegiances, developed over at least three years of training, cut across institutional boundaries (Øvretveit 1997). When the roles of other professions are poorly understood, rivalry and miscommunication become extremely likely.

- A substantial barrier to the creation of genuinely collaborative relationships with clients is created by the very lengthy professional socialization of all health professionals. D'amour et al (2005:117) state that 'Throughout their education [health professionals] are socialized to adopt a discipline-based vision of their clientele and the services they offer.'

  This, in part, is created by the inculcation of the medical model, and the associated expertise grounded in objective scientific knowledge. As we have seen in Chapter 5, there is evidence that health professionals' attitudes towards disabled people are no more enlightened than those expressed by the lay population (French 1996c). Hafferty (2006:1298) argues that this has created dilemmas for professionals in relation to partnership:

  > Recent calls for a patient-centered medicine rooted in egalitarian notions of a partnership among equals have served to heighten this tension between traditional medical authority (e.g. the physician as expert – the patient as the object of that

expertise) and the physician–patient relationship as a partnership of authoritative equals.

Thus, though professionals may ostensibly court a partnership approach, they are entrenched in a system in which their professional expertise is the very essence of their identity as professionals. Basnett (2001), a medical doctor who became disabled himself later in his career, offers a reflection on his changing view of disability once personally affected. He argues that the lengthy training of health professionals, together with their experience of working with people only when they are in need of treatment (and not when they are well or coping) means that '… health professionals can develop a view of disability that is at substantial variance from its reality for many disabled people' (Basnett 2001:451). He goes on to suggest that health, particularly medical, professionals have a vested interest in promulgating individualistic interpretations of disability as it justifies and strengthens their own role. Basnett (2001:452) states:

> It emphasises the importance of their skill and assists in their professional dominance. The need to provide interventions that cure the individual or provide psychological and physical adjustment to disability is reinforced.

- The organizational context, particularly within the NHS is highly complex. The notion of partnership relies on the co-ordination of effort among many different professional groups, each with rather different priorities, conceptual frameworks, jargons, cultures and ways of working. Mello-Baron et al (2003) argue that in the movement towards healthcare trust status there is a lack of resources and attention to partnership. They state (2003:129):

  > The professional domains remain focussed upon 'how we can work together' rather than addressing common skills and values, which may lead to a 'generic', 'hybrid' or 'doubly qualified' worker … The new welfare picture leaves users in a position of initiating, developing and maintaining links across many specialist areas.

- It is also a markedly resource-limited environment, so it is not surprising that professional groups sometimes compete with each other for the resources to do their jobs effectively. As Heywood (2006), for instance, points out, The Code of Ethics and Professional Conduct for Occupational Therapists offers specific guidance about the duty of advocacy for the client, duty to record unmet needs and duty to bring resource deficiencies to the attention of managers. It does not present an easy context for establishing effective partnership when professional agencies are each advocating for scarce resources to support their role.

- The organizational context can also impede effective relationships between service providers and users through setting up health professionals as 'gatekeepers'. This again is a resources issue, as service providers are placed in a role of rationing limited resources to clients. Inadequate budgets, for instance, may force occupational therapists to limit the provision of aids and adaptations that they know would make a great deal of difference to a client's quality of life. Given limited budgets, Heyward (2006:39) asks whether occupational therapists 'see themselves as the champion of the disabled person or as the guardian of the public purse? Or do they see themselves chiefly as the employee whose managers have given instructions and laid down guidelines that must be followed?' Nevertheless, looking from a medical model viewpoint, championing disabled people can be equated with being a guardian of the public purse. For instance, the goal of 'independence' from a medical viewpoint can be associated with lack of supposed 'special' equipment and support. Thus, independence for a disabled person can be equated with independence from resources.

- Government targets and deadlines (for instance, to reduce waiting lists) inevitably impact not only on the wider organization but also on individual encounters between a therapist and a client. For example, pressures on appointment times may encourage therapists to focus narrowly on biomedical or functional issues and to ignore the wider psychosocial problems that the client is experiencing.

- People who are powerless and marginalized within society may not be able to readily express themselves, to make complaints or to effect change. O'Sullivan (2000:86) states that:

  A principle of sound decision-making practice is for clients to have the highest feasible level of involvement, but they may not always feel sufficiently empowered to make decisions … Stakeholders need to consult with each other to share information but the presence of clients at these meetings is not sufficient in itself to ensure their involvement. Active steps may be required to prevent them being excluded from meaningful participation.

Activity 9.4

FROM THE VIEWPOINT OF DISABLED PEOPLE

The following is an extract from a report summarizing some of the views expressed in a focus group of disabled people at Derbyshire Centre for Integrated Living (taken from an unpublished research report by Swain). They were discussing the barriers they face in their daily lives. As you read make a note of the underlying issues in terms of effective partnership.

Disabled participants repeatedly referred to the attitudes of those with power over their lives and, associated with this, the presumptions that are made about themselves and their lifestyles. Relations with professionals who profess the expertise to define disabled people's needs together with being providers of the solutions, which they also control, are key to the barriers to independent living. Participants spoke of their power struggle in everyday interactions with health and social care professionals:

It's the professionals ... they do what they consider a care package but it's not a lifestyle package ... they just put what they see as your needs ... they don't see transport, they don't see social, they just see fed and watered and go to bed ... you are socially excluded because of what they perceive ...

Life's a constant battle ... they just don't see you the way they see themselves.

Most OTs have genuinely impressive knowledge of the muscular-skeletal system, but the system they work then supposes on that basis they can determine the physical, emotional, intellectual, social and spiritual needs and requirements of any person with any kind of impairment.

They purport to have the expertise.

Perhaps the first thing you might have noted is that the views expressed here concur with the views of disabled people expressed in other research projects referred to in this book. The daily barriers faced by disabled people can include coping with the service system. Ostensible solutions, it seems, can themselves become barriers to partnership particularly as conceived and initiated by professionals.

Finkelstein & Stuart (1996:171) observe that:

Disabled people and their organisations are still almost completely absent from any real decision making in the planning or delivery of services or public utilities that they may use ... Information about appropriate services then, arising out of the experience and perspective of disabled peoples' lifestyles, is very limited.

There is evidence that disabled people's views of partnership are mixed, as we shall see below. Nevertheless, research by Barnes &

Mercer (2006:170) suggests that 'the notion of "partnership" alarms some disabled people, who argue strongly that user-led organizations should maintain their distance'. The evident suspicion of entering into partnership is grounded in the regulation and surveillance by statutory mechanisms and crucial funding controls. An associated fear, fed by past experience, is the colonization of disabled people's initiatives by non-disabled service providers. The question becomes: partnership on whose terms? Beresford & Campbell (1994) take this question into an analysis of representation and representativeness. In their conclusion they state (1994:191):

> There are important questions here for service agencies. Can they reconcile schemes for user involvement and empowerment with the overall political structures within which they are set? How can such schemes avoid being marginal or tokenistic? But more important perhaps, there are questions for us. How do we make best use of such participatory opportunities? How much can we really expect to get out of them?

Their final question takes us on to the final section of this chapter.

TOWARDS PARTNERSHIP WORKING

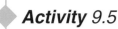

Activity 9.5

YOUR VIEWS OF POSSIBILITIES

Either from your experience in the clinical setting, or from your general observations as a service provider, draw up some possible strategies for effective partnership with service users.

Given the intransigence of the barriers to effective partnership, there is no easy route to its achievement. As with empowerment, the starting point is some general principles to provide both the foundations for developing partnership working and a framework for monitoring change:

- First, all forms of partnership are multifaceted and complex (Lymbery 2006). It is a continuing process requiring continuing critical scrutiny or reflection.

- The effective development of user involvement in partnership working must be generated by, and controlled by, service users themselves.

- The development of user involvement needs to be seen as embedded in all decision making within an organization or service, including financial and management decision making at all levels – local, regional and national.

- There is no body of concern that can be seen as 'user involvement' that is separate or isolated from partnership in all decision-making structures and processes within an organization – including finance and management.

- Partnership in policy making is crucial. Service users should be involved in the writing of policy, rather than being simply consulted about drafts of policy statements.

- Approaches to partnership working need to be open, flexible and individual (or client centred).

- Effective communication is fundamental to partnership and user involvement. This includes a creative and flexible approach to group meetings including, for instance, video conferencing.

Turning to more specific strategies and beginning at the level of service provider–user interactions, therapists need a wide variety of communication skills if they are to work in effective partnerships with service users. The following list is adapted from Reynolds (2004b):

- Listening and understanding the service user's story.
- Providing information.
- Asking questions.
- Motivating, encouraging and re-establishing hope.
- Providing feedback about progress.
- Helping the service user to challenge negative thoughts and expectations.
- Supporting the service user's decision making and control.
- Raising awareness of disabling cultural forces.

In terms of partnership encompassed within the notion of service user involvement, the literature suggests that methods of involving users of services can take many forms. For instance, Brown (2000) lists the following methods with particular reference to residential care for disabled people:

- Residents' committees.
- User panels.
- Customer surveys.
- Suggestion boxes.

- Involvement in management committees.
- Involvement in forums and working parties.
- Focus groups.
- Public meetings.

Looking towards the inclusion of all disabled people, Bewley & Glendinning (1994) warn against relying heavily on any one method, as none are perfect and a variety are needed to reach all disabled people. They state (1994:16):

> There are a range of methods by which disabled people and voluntary organisations are involved in community care planning and there is nothing necessarily inappropriate about using any of them. What disabled people involved in this project criticised was the reliance by social and health services on a small range of methods to reach and consult all disabled people on all matters; the burdens which involvement placed on individuals; the exclusion of more marginalised groups and communities; and the lack of clarity and debate about the purpose of each method and its suitability for achieving that purpose.

They note a heavy reliance on formal meetings in service-user involvement and point out that in order to reach black disabled people, people living in rural areas and other marginalized groups such as travellers and people with learning difficulties, a community development approach, working with local networks, needs to be adopted on a sustained basis. Carr (2004), in her review of the literature, found that little attention was paid to the diversity of users even though those from ethnic minorities were often in most need of services. She also found that the belief that disabled people from ethnic minorities 'look after their own' (and therefore do not need services) is still prevalent. The inequalities in health and social services that people from ethnic minority groups experience has been well documented and will be discussed further in Chapter 10.

Turning to the standpoint of disabled people, or 'service users', Beresford et al (1997) note that organizations of disabled people have influenced mainstream services by collaborating in projects and by training professionals in disability issues. Some disabled people feel that this collaboration is strategically important to ensure their involvement in community care (though, as we saw above, others are cautious). In their research into self-organized user groups of social and healthcare services, Barnes et al (1999a) found that the representation of disabled people within key decision-making forums was seen as both an end in itself and a means for achieving other objectives. One participant, for instance, stated (Barnes et al 1999a:24):

> I think the Patients' Council works well because it does work on the principle that it's not one or two of our service users ... sitting on the edge of a meeting or whatever, it is managers, senior managers coming to meet service users to be accountable and really they have to account on the spot.

As you saw in Chapter 7, a very important component of user involvement has been the development of services that are run and controlled by disabled people for disabled people. If we return to the four relationships or types of partnerships outlined in the introduction to this chapter, they can be viewed as inter-related. The partnership between disabled people themselves is a key to shifting the power relations between service providers and service users.

CONCLUSION

As a result of the changes in ideology, policy and legislation, the 1990s saw a growth in user-involvement initiatives where many disabled people now participate in a range of activities (Carmichael 2004). Few initiatives, however, have been thoroughly evaluated and many have proved ineffective (Beresford et al 1997, Carr 2004). Robson et al (2003) and Carr (2004) note the lack of research, monitoring and evaluation with regard to the impact and outcome of user participation. Professional agencies tend to focus on the benefits of participation itself rather than on the outcomes achieved, sometimes even viewing participation as a form of 'therapy' to improve the skills, competence and self-esteem of disabled people (Braye 2000, Carr 2004). It is clear that until there is a shift in power between professionals and disabled people, true partnership between them, in all its facets, will not be fully realized.

Chapter 10

How do services meet diverse needs?

WHAT'S THE DIFFERENCE?

What is meant by 'diverse needs'? The obvious starting point is that all service users have individual needs. This is the basis of client-centred approaches within therapy practice. All service users coming to therapy bring with them their particular circumstances, their specific lifestyles and their distinctive networks of support, beliefs, values, motivations and, of course, needs.

Activity 10.1

THE SOURCES OF DIVERSITY

The following is an extract from a research report (which we used in Ch. 9) that summarizes some views expressed by visually impaired service users. The extracts we have selected are relevant to understanding needs (Swain et al 2005). As you read, think about and make a list of the main factors that underlie the diversity of needs. All the participants are visually impaired service users, but how might they differ as people using services? How might their needs, too, be different from other service users'?

There are certain things that happen, like a spill of anything. It's very difficult and it's where I feel that at least once a week they should have someone either from Social Services or the Sight Service coming just to check, as a friend say, and say, 'Well this needs doing' ... I'm sure that most people would accept that.

(p. 25)

I think it makes their life easier if you fit into a check box. They need to be more dynamic in their thinking about things. In other words it has to be done on a person-to-person basis. And what they really need is somebody in the field that can take on the situation, and sadly I don't think you will find many fully sighted people who would be able to do this.

(p. 26)

I do my own cooking and everything like that. I would rather do that. When the carers came all they wanted to do was put a micro meal in or do some sandwiches, and I don't like sandwiches.

(p. 26)

I should point out that the Newcastle Society sponsors a macular disease group and I need it and we have a meeting every month here ... we have speakers and the speakers are good, very useful. But I've discovered over the years, the very important part of the meeting is the cup of tea and chat, because people are coming in who have just been registered and they are still in a state of shock and it is very useful to be able to talk to someone and hear other people's experiences and get tips and advice.

(p. 17)

And then you've got to deal with orientation round the place itself and that goes into every detail too, 'Is there a canteen?', 'Is there a loo?' ... I don't want to be led around by my work colleagues, I like to preserve my dignity.

(p. 20)

Yes, I have a care worker, Peter, nice chap. He gives me a helping hand. It's good but I only get four hours a week and it isn't enough ... I live on my own, and he is the only person I see from one end of the week to the other and I don't know what is out there in the big wide world ... we have enough time to get my shopping done and to do a bit of housework.

(p. 25)

You may have noted that the list of possible differences is seemingly endless, going back to the idea that needs are individual. Nevertheless, the following are some of the key factors, often cited as underlying diversity, which you may have noted in the quotations:

- The first sources you may have noted are associated with impairment. 'Visual impairment' is not a single condition and is not associated with one clear set of common needs. The needs of people with macular degeneration can differ from those of people with glaucoma. The needs of people whose visual impairment is deteriorating or variable can be different from those of people with a stable impairment.

- The age of onset of impairment may be significant. People born visually impaired can have different needs from people who become visually impaired in later life.

- Severity of impairment can be significant to needs.

- Type of impairment is a factor. The needs of visually impaired people can differ from people with mobility impairments, and differ again from those of people with both visual and mobility impairments.

- Looking towards the social context, the list can be added to by numerous factors. Economics and associated social class, for instance, are sources of diversity.

- Gender, ethnicity, age, sexual orientation and religion may all impact upon needs.

- Geography or locality – there can be diversity of needs depending on where service users live, for instance in an urban or rural environment.

- Finally, personal preferences reverberate throughout the diversity of needs. For instance, when I (Sally) started a new job, I was assured that somebody would always take me to wherever I had to go. I, however, found the thought of this terrible as I need to feel orientated in a place if I am to be there for any length of time. Also I did not like the thought of 'waiting around' for people. This shows the complexity of the issue because being 'taken' can be very relaxing if it happens just now and again. My feelings may be to do with how I, and my visually impaired contemporaries, were socialized, especially at special school, when, to be 'independent' (in a narrow sense) was so strongly espoused.

The topic for this chapter is, then, vast and complex. To address the relevant issues we will look first at understandings of diversity. We will concentrate on two areas: inequality, as diversity is significant in terms of social structures of power and resources; and culture, as diversity is significant in terms of the social resources service users bring to therapy. We then review the construction of diversity in health and health care. Is need randomly or unequally distributed between groups of people? From this analysis we turn to implications for services in meeting diverse needs.

UNDERSTANDING DIVERSITY

 Activity *10.2*

WHY ARE THERE DIVERSE NEEDS?

As we have begun to see, service users come into the therapy process with a wide variety of needs. Why are needs diverse? Take some time to think and make a few notes on explanations of the diversity of needs.

Perhaps the most obvious answer to the question in the above activity is that service users are individuals and have individual needs. There are, as usual however, questions behind the question. What are needs? How do they differ from other concepts such as wishes and rights? These are longstanding debates in which the whole idea of needs has come under considerable scrutiny and criticism (Swain et al 2003). One line of questioning is generated by the power relations between professionals and service users, in which professionals are dominant in defining service users' needs, particularly through assessment procedures. This has been taken a step further to question who needs needs. McKnight (1995:29) turns the concept of needs on its head to argue that it is professionals who need needs:

> Just as General Motors needs steel, a service economy *needs* 'deficiency', 'human problems' and 'needs' if it is to grow … The economic need for need creates a demand for redefining conditions of deficiency.

This is demonstrated in the history of the development of therapy services. It is evident, for instance, in the increase of services as 'needs' increased following the First and Second World Wars (see Ch. 3).

The notion of diversity can also be questioned. We could have asked you to list shared or universal needs. This is again a longstanding debate. You may be familiar with Maslow's (1954) hierarchy of needs with physiological needs at the bottom of the hierarchy, rising to safety needs, the need to be loved and to belong and, at the top, the need for self-actualization. A list of shared needs can turn us away from the nature of the individual towards the nature of humanity and society. There are physical needs, for instance for food, water, clean air, sleep and so on, interpersonal needs such as being listened to, loved and respected, and broader social needs, for instance an accessible, safe and efficient transport system, effective health care, employment and opportunities for leisure pursuits.

This notion of universal needs turns easily into notions of human rights. Citizenship rights follow from the concept of universal human needs, as without adequate levels of need satisfaction a person would be unable to fulfil his or her duties as a citizen. Thus 'all people have a strong right to need satisfaction' (Gough 1998:52). In this sense, needs can be understood in terms of human rights that are not met. Thus explanations of needs and the diversity of needs lie within the society and cultures in which we live. Understanding the diversity of needs lies in the nature of the society we create and which creates us – and our individual needs. Within social science this takes our explanation of diversity in two related directions: the cultures in which we live and the structure of (or inequalities within) society, which create and underpin the diversity of needs that therapists address daily in their practice.

The term 'culture' is the most obvious starting point in contemplating diversity, as it signifies different values, lifestyles and languages. Schein (1985:123) defines culture as:

> A set of basic assumptions – shared solutions to universal problems of external adaptation (how to survive) and internal integration (how to stay together) – which have evolved over time and are handed down from one generation to the next.

A culture, then, is a shared set of values and attitudes derived from and giving meaning to membership of and belonging to groups, and by implication non-membership of and non-belonging to other groups. Culture relates to identity and how we define who we are, and equally who we are not (Woodward 2004). In our work in the area of disability studies, we have experienced this in many manifestations expressed in different ways. Non-disabled people can, for instance, affirm their identity as 'not one of those', that is, not a member of a group identified as being disabled. But also disabled people can positively affirm their identity as 'not one of those', that is, not a non-disabled person, and in so doing challenge stereotypical views of disabled people as 'tragic'. Writing of disability culture, Vasey (2004:106) states:

> If a disabled person needs help with eating, or crossing the road, or getting up in the morning, this is part of their cultural experience. If a person gets around in a wheelchair, reads Braille or uses sign language, this is also part of their cultural experience and their way

of being. The identification of these aspects of an impaired person's life ... [is] a breakthrough in the struggle for the legitimacy of impairment and the impaired person's right to have a fair crack at life along with everybody else.

Looking towards the structures in our society, social hierarchies are manifested and maintained in many ways, for instance through racism, disablism, sexism, classism, homophobia and ageism. Those without power are marginalized and excluded from the lifestyles and quality of life enjoyed by prosperous and elite groups. Questions of inequality pervade understandings of identity, health and illness, and the provision of human services, including therapy. Let us begin with a parade.

Drawing on an original idea by Jan Penn, a Dutch economist, Macintosh & Mooney (2000) graphically describe the unequal distribution of incomes in the UK as an 'income parade'. Imagine that the total population of the UK, all 60 million, are lined up and rush past you, taking just one hour from start to finish. Imagine too that the height of the people in the parade matches their household income, so that the greater the person's household income the taller he or she is. The average height of the people in the parade is 5 ft 8 in and this is the height of the couples with an average household income (statistics taken from the early 1990s). So, here they come racing past, from the shortest (the poorest) to the tallest (the richest). After 3 minutes a single unemployed mother of two children passes by. She is living below the government's income support level and is 1 ft 10 in tall. Everyone who passes in the first 12 minutes has less than half the average income and so are less than 2 ft 10 in tall. After 21 minutes the couple passing by are a full-time vehicle exhaust fitter and his wife who is not in paid employment. They are 3 ft 9 in tall. After half an hour, with half the population having passed you, it may surprise you that the people passing are not of average height. They are only 4 ft 10 in tall with a household income that is just 83% of the national average. When do people with an average household income pass by? Those of average height, with average income, do not pass you until 62% of the population have passed by, but to understand why this is we need to look to the end of the parade. After three-quarters of an hour the people are getting taller, about 6 ft 10 in now, but it is not until the last ten minutes that the height of the people passing really begins to grow. With three minutes left the couple passing are 11 ft 11 in tall. They are in their late fifties and their children have left home. He is a self-employed freelance journalist and she is a part-time manager of an old people's day centre. In the last minute a company chief executive and his wife, who is not in paid employment, pass by. They are both at least 60 ft high. It is in the last seconds that the real giants arrive, people whose heights can be measured in miles, the richest being at least 4 miles high.

We think this graphically illustrates economic inequality, from being less than 2 ft tall to having your head in the clouds. Evidence also suggests that this gap is widening. Definitions of poverty are disputed. A common measure, however, is a household income at or below 60% of the national average (those passing by in the income parade for the first 12 minutes). In the UK the number of people living in poverty rose from 5 million to 13.9 million in the years between 1979 and 1991–1992. In 2004/2005 11.4 million people lived below the poverty threshold, including 3.4 million children. This demonstrates a drop of 2.5 million since 1996/1967 but is much higher than in the early 1980s (www.poverty.org.uk).

Poverty, however it is defined, is not simply a matter of lack of financial resources as in the income parade. There are, as Thompson (1998:91) suggests, significant social implications in terms of:

- psychological wellbeing, particularly in relation to self-esteem
- social relations – low income groups can be marginalized or excluded in certain social situations
- insecurity – economic deprivation can make it difficult, if not impossible, to plan ahead or develop a 'life plan'
- access to resources and services – for example health and education.

To this list we would add the prevention of full participation in contemporary culture, through the lack of resources and technology this requires.

So what about the 'client parade', that is the line-up of clients who pass through therapy? What would the parade of clients who passed through therapy last year look like? Perhaps you might like to imagine them passing by you in an hour-long parade! The statistics are not available, though it is highly unlikely that the client parade is a simple reflection, or random sample, from the income parade. One important factor in the client parade is the distribution of health problems and it is to inequalities in health that we turn next.

DIVERSITY IN HEALTH AND HEALTH CARE

A key question in relation to diverse needs is whether health is randomly distributed: can illness strike anyone at any time irrespective of her or his income, ethnicity or gender? The overwhelming evidence suggests an unequal distribution. In most countries of the world there are large inequalities in health, with those people with the lowest socio-economic status having the worst health. Certain groups within society such as women, old people, people from ethnic minorities and disabled people are disadvantaged partly because of their over-representation in the lower socio-economic groups. There are also regional variations in health status (Talley 2004). Furthermore, in Britain as in most countries of the Western world, these inequalities are increasing (Department of Health 2001, Talley 2004). Benzeval et al (1995a:1) state that:

> It is one of the greatest contemporary social injustices that people who live in the most disadvantaged circumstances have more illness, more disability and shorter lives than those who are more affluent. In Britain death rates at most ages are two to three times higher among the growing number of disadvantaged people than they are for their better off counterparts. Most of the main causes of death contribute to these differences and together they can reduce life expectancy by as much as eight years.

Despite various individual influences on our health, the evidence overwhelmingly suggests that broad social factors concerning housing, income, educational level, employment and social integration are far more important than our individual behaviour or medical practice and advances (Ewles & Simmett 2003).

People of the lowest socio-economic status are at far higher risk, not only of physical illness and early death, but also of accidents, premature births, mental illness and suicide (Talley 2004). There is a clear relationship between health and income that is well established and widely acknowledged. Beyond this, however, the usefulness of a simple cause–effect relationship between one risk factor and one type of disease has been extensively questioned (Atkin et al 2004). A multifactorial explanation of ill health is predominant in reviews and analyses of research. Helman (2000) lists 25 cultural factors that can be causal, contributory or protective in relation to ill health. Important here is the notion that cultural factors, diet being an obvious example, may protect against ill health as well as being a possible risk factor. Ewles & Simmett (2003:16) contend that, despite considerable effort, inequalities in health remain prominent:

> As we stand now at the beginning of the 21st century, we have developed considerable understanding of what affects people's health, and we have national and international strategies for health, which are reviewed and revised on an ongoing basis.

There is a stronger local and national emphasis on prevention, health improvement and reducing inequalities ... health issues feature more in public policy debate at both central and local government and in the health service ... But as yet it is too soon to see whether these positive developments will successfully narrow the health gap between more prosperous people and disadvantaged people in the UK today. The reality in the UK is that we are still faced with entrenched inequalities in health status, and huge problems of poverty, unemployment and homelessness. This raises questions about the distribution of wealth in society and demonstrates the extent to which health is a political issue.

The general health of people from ethnic minority communities in Britain is poorer than the indigenous white Anglo-Saxon population. Smaje (1996) suggests five cultural factors as playing a role in multifactorial causality: genetics; migration; material disadvantage; lifestyle, social networks and kinship; and racism. In relation to genetics, there are a number of disorders that mainly affect people from specific ethnic minority groups. Sickle cell disorder, for instance, is one of Britain's most common genetic diseases, affecting about 15 000 people. It largely affects African and African-Caribbean people, though it is also present in people of Mediterranean, Asian and Arab origin (Anionwu & Atkin 2001). Anionwu & Atkin make the point that sickle cell anaemia is under-resourced when compared with cystic fibrosis, which is the most common genetic disorder affecting white people in the UK.

Turning to the provision of services, there is no obvious correlation between health care and health status in any population, indeed the health service has sometimes been referred to as an 'ill health' service as it tends to respond when the damage has been done. Benzeval et al (1995b:95) state:

> There is little evidence that variations in the quantity and quality of health services between advanced industrial countries make a substantial difference to crude measures of health such as national mortality rates ... Levels of well-being and life expectancy are more closely related to the availability of decent social security, housing, employment and education than health care.

This is not to imply that inequalities in health and healthcare facilities should be tolerated. There are still many people in Britain who do not fully benefit from the facilities of the NHS. People from ethnic minorities are not well served (Atkin et al 2004) nor are people with learning difficulties (Shaughnessy & Cruse 2001). This is due to a variety of factors that include poor communication, racism, disablism and lack of cultural sensitivity. Fox & Benzeval (1995) believe that an important role of the NHS should be to encourage social equity across all public departments and policies that have an impact on health. Despite the individualistic stance of most health policy, the present Labour government has taken some heed of the social determinants of health in, for example, attempting to improve education, housing and transport (Department of Health 1999). The enactment of such a change would involve an increase in services such as outreach, the mobilization of self-help groups and community action. At a broader level it would mean involvement in areas such as housing, employment, education, leisure and community regeneration (Ewles & Simmett 2003). Such a development would move health professionals from their role as clinical practitioners dealing with the consequences of ill health, to the broader arena of health promotion and political activism.

The documented views of black disabled people consistently speak of experiences of segregation and marginalization within services. For instance, in their research into the views and experiences of young black disabled people, Bignall & Butt (2000) report feelings of segregation due to racism in settings segregated due to disablism. Summarizing the evidence from several studies, Butt & Mirza (1996:94) state:

> The fact that major surveys of the experience of disability persist in hardly mentioning the experience of black disabled people should not deter us from appreciating the messages that emerge from existing work. Racism, sexism and disablism intermingle to amplify the need for supportive social care. However these same factors sometimes mean that black disabled people and their carers get a less than adequate service.

In their study of young black disabled people's experiences and views, Bignall & Butt (2000:49) conclude:

> Our interviews revealed that most of these young people did not have the relevant information to help them achieve independence. Hardly any knew of new provisions, such as Direct Payments, which would help with independent living. Most people did not know where to get help or information they wanted, for example, to move into their own place or go to university.

It is clear that the understanding of diverse needs requires a very broad perspective on the meaning of health, illness and disability as well as an appreciation of how age, gender, ethnicity and other social divisions can impact on health and the health care received.

TOWARDS MEETING DIVERSE NEEDS

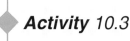

Activity 10.3

HOW TO MEET DIVERSE NEEDS

As we have seen, critical reflection is generated by 'what' questions (sources of diverse needs) and 'why' questions (explanations of diversity). We turn next to the implications for policy, provision and practice and the core question set by the title of this chapter: how do services meet diverse needs? From your knowledge and experience of therapy list the main strategies for meeting diverse needs.

Looking towards the general literature and developments in this arena, there are a number of notions that may relate to your list, including equal opportunities, equality training, inclusive practice, multiculturism, and anti-racist and anti-sexist practice. We have selected just three to examine in more depth: anti-discriminatory practice, equality training and inclusive practice.

Anti-discriminatory practice recognizes the difference of class, sexual orientation and other social divisions as the fabric of individual differences. Indeed anti-discriminatory and anti-oppressive practice are often used as umbrella terms that incorporate challenging dominant ideologies and strategies for empowerment. Braye & Preston-Shoot (1995) differentiate between anti-discriminatory and anti-oppressive practice. In their model, anti-discriminatory practice is reformist and challenges inequality within officially sanctioned rules, procedures and structures. Specific strategies include equal access to services, ethnically sensitive services and consultation about services. Anti-oppressive practice, in this model, seeks more fundamental changes in power structures. Specific strategies include rebalancing power relationships between professionals and clients, with client control of services and resources and identification and challenging abuses of power experienced by clients. In most of the literature, however, the two terms are used interchangeably, though similar ideas are used.

Thompson (2001:162) points out that 'establishing a basis of equality and social justice in service provision is no easy matter'. In the face of different forms of discrimination and multiple discrimination, and also the vested power interests that obstruct change, there can be no simple formulaic solutions to developing the practice of health professionals.

Successful change will depend on collective commitment and action. Questioning dominant racist ideologies involves actively seeking aware-ness and understanding of our own racism and that of others; examining ways in which our attitudes, understandings and behaviour contribute to racism; and challenging and seeking to avoid cultural and racial stereo-typing. The issues are further complicated when it is recognized that such stereotyping does not solely refer to the attitudes of white people. There can, of course, be stereotyping between, for instance, African-Caribbean and Asian people. Therapists wishing to challenge racism in their organ-izations need to begin along two lines suggested by Dominelli (1997:146):

> The first is that they subject their work to being monitored and evaluated by black people. The second is that they form anti-racist collectives ... sharing their anti-racist objectives and develop ways of working together and supporting each other.

It is essential that the 'voice' of clients, individual and collective, directs the provision of appropriate and culturally sensitive services. This applies through listening to individual clients whose daily experiences are likely to be fundamentally different from the experiences of health-care professionals. It also applies through the consultation of organiza-tions of people, such as people with learning difficulties and people from ethnic minority communities, at every stage of service planning and implementation.

The employment of disabled, ethnic minority staff is of crucial importance. The discrimination faced by clients from minority groups can be faced too by members of staff and people from minority groups seeking employment, highlighting the importance of equal oppor-tunity and anti-discriminatory policies. There are many advantages to the employment of staff from minority groups. Ethnic minority staff, for instance, can communicate with clients in their own languages and can contribute to the evaluation of the adequacy of services, though it is important that such staff do not become restricted in their role to 'race experts' (Dominelli 2002).

'Ethnic matching' has been a widely debated and contested strategy in the management of provision of services for minority groups. Taking a specific focus on sickle cell anaemia and thalassaemia counsellors, for instance, Anionwu (1996:184) argues that 'Those involved in recruiting candidates to these posts should actively seek out applicants from rele-vant ethnic groups from their local community'. On a wider front, how-ever, the issues are complex and multiple. Shifting the debate to disability, it can be argued that disabled service practitioners will have more sensitivity towards, and a better understanding of, the experiences of disabled service users. There are, however, questions relating to specific impairments: for instance, the understanding and sensitivity of a service provider with a visual impairment towards service users with learning difficulties. From a service provider's viewpoint, another issue is the presumptions and career limitations of being channelled to work with particular groups of service users, as we touched upon in Chapter 6.

So far in this section on 'how', we have looked at anti-discriminatory practice. We turn finally to process and concentrate on the provision of an inclusive communication environment. Here the question of how to meet diverse needs lies in the communication between therapists and service users. As with empowerment, the meeting of diverse needs is addressed through a set of principles underlying practice. Again, principles are ideals towards which therapy practice is directed and against which practice is reflected upon (Swain et al 2004a). Here we shall suggest just five.

Participation

Priority needs to be given to the participation of service users in the planning and evaluation of changing policy, provision and practice in developing inclusive communication. The onus is on service providers to face the challenges of enabling true participation of service users in decision-making processes, recognizing that service users need to participate in different ways. These include the democratic representation of the views of organizations of service users. Participation also includes as wide a consultation process as possible. Service users often continue to be treated as passively dependent on the expertise of others, yet control seems to have become increasingly central to social change for service users. A disabled person interviewed by French (2004:106) put it succinctly:

> Users should have more power. Until you give users real power, real control we'll get nowhere … there's an awful lot of people with a lot of vested interests. The more we shout about rights the more people get afraid. I'd like to see therapy training following the social model rather than the medical model. The only way to do it is to get much more input from disabled people into the training.

Accessible communication

The issues around language and ethnicity are complex but there are many examples of good practice. The Sandwell Integrated Language and Communication Service (SILCS) in the West Midlands involves a range of local health organizations – health authorities, NHS Direct, primary care groups, local authorities and voluntary agencies – working together to provide a pooled resource for spoken, written and telephone translation and interpreting, as well as sign language interpreters (Douglas et al 2004). Accessibility of communication, however, needs management beyond such a resource, including training for staff on using interpreters. The provision of written information in a range of languages must ensure that translations meet the information needs of ethnic minority communities and are culturally relevant. There are, of course, many social factors within the diversity of the needs of people from ethnic minority communities. As Dominelli (1997:107) argues, for instance, 'translation services should be publicly funded and provide interpreters matched to clients' ethnic grouping, language, religion, class and gender'.

Much is known about the accessibility of information based on the views expressed by disabled people. Clark (2002) offers wide ranging recommendations which cover such things as alternative formats. He states 'the following formats should be available – large print, large print with pictures and symbols, Braille, computer disc containing the file in plain text format, accessible websites, audiotape, videotape with plain, spoken language, audio description and British Sign Language' (Clark 2002:62).

For some people, particularly those with communication disabilities, the issue of time can be crucial to inclusive communication environments. For people with communication disabilities a slower tempo can be the only accessible pace to ensure understanding. A participant within research by Knight et al (2002:17) explains:

> I would rather repeat myself ten times than have someone finish a sentence for me. This is why I won't use a communication aid.
>
> I prefer to speak for myself and I would rather repeat myself several times than have someone say they understood me when they did not.

Along similar lines, Pound & Hewitt (2004) emphasize that the speed of communication and the length of meetings need careful consideration if people with communication impairments are to be included successfully.

Diversity and flexibility

Douglas et al (2004:74) point to some of the complexities when attempting to respect diversity and provide flexible services:

> Interpreting is extremely complex in that interpreters must ensure that the patient or client easily understands the language they use. Again other factors, such as class, region, religion and geography,

may impinge on the process of interpreting and communication – such that just speaking the same language may not necessarily mean the same understanding will follow.

The lists of recommendations for communication access, as produced by Clark (2002) and others, clearly challenge the imperatives of normality and emphasize the diversity of communication styles and formats. Nevertheless, there are diverse needs even within specific groups of people with impairments, which again puts the emphasis on listening to and control by individual people. As a person with a visual impairment, I (Sally) have found, for example, that I am often presented with large print even though it is the depth, font and colour contrast that are more important to me.

Human relations

Communication is constructed and embedded in relationships between people. The notion of personal relationships can be seen as irrevocably intertwined with communication. Communication is a means of expressing a relationship: it constitutes the initiation, maintenance and ending of a relationship; and it is the medium and substance through which the relationship is defined and given meaning. A disabled client offered advice to therapists on the basis of her experience (French 2004:103):

> Forget you're a therapist – just be yourself. I don't mean forget all your training – but be yourself. Don't be afraid of showing the real you because that's what makes people respond, when they're ill they respond more easily if the therapist is being real.

Use of inclusive language

In part this reflects the idea that language controls or constructs thinking. Sexism, ageism, homophobia, racism and disablism are framed within the very language we use. This has been characterized and degraded by some people as 'political correctness' (PC), often with reference to examples that seem trivial or fatuous (for example, being criticized for offering black or white coffee). Use of language, however, is not simply about the legitimacy of words or phrases – what we are allowed to say or not say. As Thompson (1998) explains, language is a powerful vehicle within interactions between health and social care professionals and clients. He identifies a number of key issues:

1. Jargon – the use of specialized language, creating barriers and mystification and reinforcing power differences.

2. Stereotypes – terms used to refer to people that reinforce presumptions, for example disabled people as 'sufferers'.

3. Stigma – terms that are derogatory and insulting, for example 'mentally handicapped'.

4. Exclusion – terms that exclude, overlook or marginalize certain groups, for example the term 'Christian name'.

5. Depersonalization – terms that are reductionist and dehumanizing, for example 'the elderly', 'the disabled' and even 'CPs' (to denote people with cerebral palsy).

In this light, questions of the use of language go well beyond listing acceptable and unacceptable words and include examining ways of thinking that rationalize, legitimize and underline unequal professional–client power relations.

CONCLUSION

 Activity 10.4

HOW TO MEET DIVERSE NEEDS MORE EFFECTIVELY

Return to the list of strategies for meeting diverse needs you put together for Activity 10.3. Again, from your knowledge and experience list the main ways in which these strategies could be improved in the situation in which you work or have worked as a therapist or a student.

We hope the ideas in the previous section of this chapter provided some food for thought. Meeting diverse needs within health care is central to the provision of services, and creates complex tasks for all therapists and the managers of organizations in which they work. Communication beyond listening, however important that may be, is required. Therapists need a full appreciation of cultural identity and structural inequalities if the services they provide are to respect every person as a unique individual with skills, insight and knowledge to bring to the professional–client encounter.

Chapter **11**

How do professionals find out?

In this chapter we will be considering research within physiotherapy and occupational therapy. Research is of fundamental importance to therapy students and practising physiotherapists and occupational therapists for numerous reasons – from the requirement on students to conduct small-scale projects to the general pursuit of evidence-based practice. We focus on a shift of thinking in research that is centrally concerned with the relations between those who conduct research and those who are research subjects. The crucial shift is from doing research *on* people to doing research *with* people. This is not to suggest that participatory research (research *with* people) is the only approach that is of value within physiotherapy and occupational therapy. It is rather a shift within social science research generally that challenges thinking within therapy research and offers possible alternatives to more traditional approaches. In this chapter we will concentrate specifically on research in the field of disability while recognizing that the general principles have a wider application.

The chapter begins with an overview of the development of participatory research, what this shift in thinking is, and why researchers have moved towards this approach. We then turn to disability research and discuss why disabled people are dissatisfied with research done *on* them. In this context we look at what has come to be known as emancipatory research and contrast this with participatory research to pinpoint key issues for researchers and disabled people. We then highlight examples of research with disabled people that involves them and gives their perspective and, finally, we will consider the implications of this for physiotherapists and occupational therapists.

Activity 11.1

WHO MAKES DECISIONS IN RESEARCH?

Think about a research project within occupational therapy or physiotherapy with which you have been involved or one that you have heard or read about. What was the role of the research subjects in the project? What was the purpose of the research and who, if anyone, do you think benefited from it? Who chose the research topic and the research methods to be used and who decided how the research would be conducted and disseminated?

We do not know which research project you chose to consider but unless it was conducted in very recent times it is likely that the research subjects had little part to play in the process apart from providing the data by, for instance, filling in questionnaires, being interviewed or taking part in an experiment. With regard to who benefited, it is likely that the researcher benefited more than the research subjects in terms of qualifications, pay, promotion and prestige. The researcher is also likely to have made all of the decisions about what to research, which methodologies to use and how and where to disseminate the findings. We will be discussing these issues in more detail later in the chapter. It is important to realize at this point that research findings, however convincing, do not automatically influence practice as research is enmeshed within social, cultural and political processes. You may like to reflect on how far physiotherapy and occupational therapy practice is based upon research evidence.

RESEARCH WITH PEOPLE

Brechin (1993:73) states that research '… tends to be owned and controlled by researchers, or by those who, in turn, own and control the researchers', for instance those who provide the funding. Researchers who adopt a participatory approach are attempting to change these power relations and to ensure that research is owned and controlled by research participants as well as researchers. In characterizing participatory research, Cornwell & Jewkes (1995:1667) argue that, '... the key differ-ence between participatory and conventional methodologies lies in the location of power in the research process'. You will note that within participatory research the language has changed from 'subjects' to 'par-ticipants' to reflect this orientation.

Participatory methodologies have arisen from qualitative research approaches which aim to reflect, explore and disseminate the views, concerns, feelings and experiences of research participants from their own perspective. The aim of participatory research goes beyond this, how-ever, to engage participants in the design, conduct and evaluation of research within non-hierarchical research relations (Zarb 1992). Feminist research has been particularly influential in this development where the objection has been that male researchers have spoken on behalf of women (Walmsley & Johnson 2003). Participatory research can also be viewed as an aspect of wider changes within health and social care and society generally. These include the development of user involvement, consumer participation and empowerment (French & Swain in press, Kemshall & Littlechild 2000) along with a lessening of deference towards 'experts' and an unquestioning belief in their knowledge and skills (Chafetz 1996, McKnight 1995).

As noted above, a crucial tenet of participatory research is that it is research *with* rather than *on* people (Reason & Heron 1986). The research process is viewed as a potential source of change and empowerment for the research participants as well as a process for influencing professional policy and practice by reflecting the views and opinions of service users. Reason & Heron (1986) believe that participatory research invites people to concur in the co-creation of knowledge about themselves, which is achieved by their active involvement at every stage of the research process – from choice of topic to evaluation and dissemination of the findings. Chambers (1997), talking of participatory research within developing countries, identified the following key features:

- It breaks down the mystique surrounding research.
- It ensures that the problems researched are perceived as problems by the community to which the research is directed.
- It helps to develop self-confidence, self-reliance and skills within the research participants.
- It encourages democratic interaction and transfer of power to the research participants.

Participatory research is thus essentially about establishing equality in research relationships.

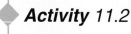

Activity 11.2

THE BARRIERS TO INVOLVEMENT IN RESEARCH

Jot down any examples you can think of in physiotherapy and occupational therapy research where the involvement of disabled people extends beyond the role of research participants. What, in your view, are the barriers to involving research participants more fully in therapy research?

Involving research participants in wider aspects of the research process is a relatively recent development. You may have come across research of this type in recent therapy books and journals – we offer a few examples at the end of the chapter. The barriers to the fuller involvement of disabled people in the research process are numerous. They include practical barriers such as time and funding, and attitudinal barriers such as disbelief that disabled people are sufficiently 'expert' to be valid researchers or to have a sound and authoritative perspective. Indeed the perspective that disabled people have may feel threatening and be rejected by other people. This is explored in the following activity.

Activity 11.3

THE VOICE OF DISABLED PEOPLE IN RESEARCH

It is only in very recent times that the voices of disabled people and other marginalized groups have been heard within research. This started to happen with the development of qualitative research approaches. In a very early qualitative study, Mills (in 1962, cited in Pilgrim & Rogers 1999) interviewed users of mental health care services. This research uncovered that they preferred contact with non-professionals to professionals and that they derived most of their support from 'ordinary' people such as home helps. However, in a review of this work, Jones (in 1962, cited in Pilgrim & Rogers 1999:343) wrote:

It is hard to believe that there were no sympathetic and sensible social workers in the area ... The material is taken very largely from patients and their relatives and no attempt at validation appears to have been made. Since some of the patients were suffering from paranoia, and others from depression, it would have been a basic precaution to check the objective value of statements with the medical records or the responsible psychiatrist.

What does this quotation tell you about the place of disabled and other marginalized people in research at this time? What repercussions might there have been?

It is clear from this quotation that the users of the mental health care services and their relatives were not believed by those in power. Their views were disregarded and were thought to be far less reliable than those of the professionals. Research always takes place within a political context and it is likely that the health and social care professionals would have been affronted by these findings and would have striven to suppress them or, more likely, just ignored them. As we have seen in previous chapters, failing to ask disabled people for their views, and to take them seriously, has meant that policies and services have been built and delivered in inappropriate and abusive ways. Talking of people with learning disabilities, Walmsley & Johnson (2003:126) state:

> History shows that medicine and positivist research has objectified them, pursued goals which set them apart from the rest of humanity and has often led to oppressive policies directed towards them. Work around IQ testing in the early twentieth century falls into this category as do many current studies of 'challenging behaviour' … We believe that as researchers we have a responsibility to people with learning disabilities not to add to this history.

Sometimes disabled people have been considered too vulnerable to take part in research, and in that way have been silenced, or funding for research which explores disabled peoples' lives or opinions may be difficult to obtain (French et al 2001).

We undertook a brief content analysis of the peer reviewed articles in the UK journal *Physiotherapy* from January 1999 to December 2001 (French & Swain 2004). This revealed that, with regard to research studies of patients and clients, the experimental method was three times more common than the summed total of qualitative and survey methods. Qualitative and survey methods which focused on healthcare professionals (where, for example, their opinions and feelings were sought) were over three times as common as those which focused on the opinions and feelings of patients and clients. Twelve case studies and five studies using a documentary method were published during this period. All of these studies showed a strong biomedical and quantitative orientation. Psychological, social and cultural perspectives were minor compared with the biomedical perspective, while the perspective of the disabled people's movement was entirely absent. This indicates the dominance of biomedical knowledge within physiotherapy, derived from experimental research, and the marginalization of other sources of knowledge, including the direct voice of disabled people themselves.

***Activity** 11.4*

UNCOVERING TRENDS IN THERAPY RESEARCH

Conduct a similar content analysis on a more recent sample of physiotherapy and occupational therapy journals. Do the trends that we discovered persist and do they generalize to other occupational therapy and physiotherapy journals? Has the situation changed in recent years?

Research is not justifiable simply on the traditional grounds of furthering knowledge with the presumption that knowledge is intrinsically good. All research is political and research production and processes can further the oppression of those who are the subjects of research. Research into the treatment of a particular disease, for instance, may serve to maintain the status quo by failing to address the social, economic and political factors involved in its aetiology. Likewise the predominance of a medical orientation in research (genetic research, for instance) has the potential to lead to abuse and oppression. Qualitative research is not immune from abusive tendencies either and researchers need to justify very clearly why they wish to investigate the lives of marginalized people, especially if the area of investigation is sensitive, for instance sexual behaviour.

DISABILITY RESEARCH

In 1992, Oliver laid down the gauntlet to researchers in the field of disability studies. He stated (1992:106):

> As disabled people have increasingly analysed their segregation, inequality and poverty in terms of discrimination and oppression, research has been seen as part of the problem rather than part of the solution … Disabled people have come to see research as a violation of their experiences, as irrelevant to their needs and as failing to improve their material circumstances and quality of life.

Disability has generally been defined in an individualistic, medicalized way as an internal condition of the individual, and most research on disability, including the government's large Office of Population Censuses and Surveys (OPCS) reflects this orientation. Many disabled people, on the other hand, view disability in terms of social, physical and attitudinal barriers which could be removed if only the political will to do so was present (Swain et al 2004b).

If an individualistic stance is taken by researchers, then the questions posed will be based on impairment and not on discriminatory practices and lack of access. Oliver has reworded some of the questions used in an OPCS survey to illustrate this point. For example, in place of the question, 'What complaint causes your difficulty in holding, gripping and turning things?' he substitutes the question, 'What defects in the design of everyday equipment, like jars, bottles and tins, cause your difficulty in holding, gripping and turning them?' and in place of the question, 'Did you move here because of your health problems/disability?' he writes, 'What inadequacies in your housing caused you to move here?' (Oliver 1990:7). Abberley (1992:158) believes that 'It is a political decision, conscious or otherwise, to employ questions of the first type rather than the second'. Medical and academic perceptions and interests have dominated disability research to the extent that the work of the researchers has barely been questioned. Whalley Hammell (2006:171) states, 'Rehabilitation researchers' good intentions appear to have been so taken for granted that little attention has been given to the nature of their work'.

As noted in previous chapters, the way in which disability is understood is a serious issue as these ideas can be translated into practice which impacts on every aspect of disabled people's lives.

◆ *Activity* *11.5*

RESEARCHERS' ATTITUDES TO DISABILITY

I (John) was involved as a research subject in a trial of a newly developed form of insulin where people with diabetes were required to complete a questionnaire about 'you and your diabetes ... the way you feel and how diabetes affects your day-to-day life'. With each question was a choice of four answers ranging from 'very much' to 'not at all'. Below are listed some of the questions

- Do you look forward to the future?
- Do you throw things around if you get upset or lose your temper?
- Do you get touchy or moody about diabetes?
- Do you hurt yourself or feel like hurting yourself when you get upset?
- Do you, even for a moment, wish that you were dead?
- Do you wish that you had never been born?

Other questions contained words such as 'fear', 'edgy', 'worry' and 'difficult'.

From reading these questions, what do you consider the researchers' underlying attitudes to diabetes are, and how far do you think this would have shaped the information obtained? If people with diabetes had been involved in this research (other than as subjects) do you think the questionnaire would have had a different orientation and, if so, in what way?

This example of research clearly demonstrates an individualistic, tragedy model of disability – although the insulin itself was successful in providing better control of John's blood sugar levels. The first question implies that the supposed tragedy of diabetes may negate any hope for the future and the following three questions focus on possible psychological responses to this tragedy. The last two questions go as far as implying that death may be preferable to having diabetes. We would suggest that the agenda within the research is clearly that of the researchers, and does not reflect the concerns of people with diabetes. For instance, the causes of any anger are clearly conceived in terms of the person's response to impairment, not the barriers faced within a disabling society (or, indeed, completing a questionnaire of this kind). It is likely that if people with diabetes had been involved in constructing the questionnaire the questions would have had a more social and environmental orientation and would have been less 'tragic'. Beeton (in press) notes that health professionals tend to underestimate the quality of life of disabled people and Whalley Hammell (2006:167) states that, '… researchers of all methodological persuasions have consistently misunderstood and distorted both the phenomenon of disability and the experience of disabled people'.

A further criticism of disability research is that most of the benefits go to the researchers rather than to disabled people themselves (Barnes 2004, Walmsley & Johnson 2003). Indeed Barnes et al (1999b) accuse researchers of being 'academic tourists' who use disability as a way of enhancing their career prospects, lifestyle and status. Disabled people have complained that researchers use them to gather information and then disappear without trace (French & Swain in press). Similar complaints have been raised by women (researchers have typically been men) and poor people in developing countries who have been investigated by Western researchers. This situation is compounded by the reluctance of funders to sponsor participatory research and to provide the extra resources that involving disabled people entails (Barnes & Mercer 2006, Walmsley & Johnson 2003).

Since the early 1990s the way in which disability has been researched has become a major issue for disabled people and their organizations. This is reflected in the importance it is given within the disability studies literature. In 1992 the Joseph Rowntree Foundation sponsored a series of seminars to discuss the issues of researching disability that culminated in a conference and a special edition of the journal *Disability, Handicap and Society* (now *Disability and Society*). There are now many chapters, articles and books on the topic of researching disability (see, for example, Barnes & Mercer 2004, Barnes & Mercer 1997, Moore et al 1998, Rioux & Bach 1994, Walmsley & Johnson 2003).

RESEARCH APPROACHES AND QUESTIONS OF POWER

So far in this chapter we have discussed the meaning of participatory research. Participatory approaches have arisen from qualitative methodologies which have been developed by non-disabled researchers who wish to break down the traditional hierarchical researcher–researched relationship. It is important to understand that the roots of participatory research lie in the development of research methodology itself, rather than the development of a different understanding of disability. Qualitative research is primarily concerned with meaning, interpretation and giving research participants 'a right of voice'. There is a commitment to seeing 'through the eyes' of research participants and a belief that social behaviour cannot be grasped until the researcher has understood the symbolic world of the research participants. Furthermore researchers in the qualitative tradition accept that the research in which they are engaged cannot be independent of their own values and perspectives. Participatory research reflects the concerns and views of disabled people but is not inherently associated with a social model of disability. As Oliver (1997:26) states, '… participatory and action research is about improving the existing social and material relations of research production; not challenging and ultimately eradicating them'.

Emancipatory research, in the area of disability at least, has its roots in the growth of the disabled people's movement and is underpinned by the social model of disability. It can be argued that emancipatory research, unlike participatory research, is not a research methodology as such but rather part of the struggle of disabled people to control the decision-making processes that shape their lives and to achieve full citizenship. As Barton (1998:38) states, 'The task of changing the social relations and conditions of research production is to be viewed as part of the wider struggle to remove all forms of oppression and discrimination in the pursuit of an inclusive society'.

Emancipatory research goes further than participatory research by aiming to change the social relations of research production, with disabled people taking complete control of the research process. The production of research within an emancipatory paradigm is viewed as part of the liberation of disabled people; that is, part of the process of empowering them and changing society. Barnes (1992:122) explains:

> Emancipatory research is about the systematic demystification of the structures and processes which create disability and the establishment of a workable 'dialogue' between the research community and disabled people in order to facilitate the latter's empowerment. To do this researchers must learn how to put their knowledge and skills at the disposal of disabled people.

He goes on to say (Barnes 2004:48):

> ... the emancipatory research agenda is about nothing less than the transformation of the material and social relations of research production. This means that in contrast to traditional approaches, disabled people and their organisations, rather than professional academics and researchers, should have control of the research process including project finance and the research agenda.

Barnes (2001) argues that accountability to the disabled community is a key component of emancipatory research and that the outcomes of the research must be meaningful to disabled people. All methods and strategies for gathering data are suitable provided they are placed firmly within an environmental and cultural context that highlights the consequences of a disabling society. As Oliver (1996:143) states, '... what should be researched is ... the disablement ingrained in the individualistic consciousness and institutionalised practices of what is, ultimately, a disablist society'. Barnes (2004) believes that doing emancipatory research cannot be conceived in terms of a single project or even a collection of projects, but is a continuous process towards the empowerment of disabled people. Zarb (1992:128) sums up the fundamental difference between participatory and emancipatory research as follows:

> Participatory research which involves disabled people in a meaningful way is perhaps a prerequisite to emancipatory research in the sense that researchers can learn from disabled people and *vice versa*, and that it paves the way for researchers to make themselves 'available' to disabled people – but it is no more than that. Simply increasing participation and involvement will never by itself constitute emancipatory research unless and until it is disabled

people themselves who are controlling the research and deciding who should be involved and how.

Although certain features of participatory and emancipatory research may overlap, one common confusion is the equating of emancipatory research with the qualitative paradigm. As noted above, there is no reason inherent within the nature of emancipatory research why it should adopt a qualitative methodology, provided the research agenda is generated by disabled people themselves. Indeed, it could be argued that a quantitative approach is more likely. For instance, emancipatory research into accessible housing for disabled people is likely to take the form of a quantitative survey to produce statistics to influence housing policies. Research undertaken at the Policy Studies Institute – Measuring Barriers within Society, for instance, aimed to make a systematic analysis of physical, social, economic and political barriers using both qualitative and quantitative measures (Zarb 1995). Similarly research into direct payments by Zarb & Nadash (1994) drew heavily on quantitative data.

The outcomes of emancipatory research are far from certain and the effectiveness of such research can only be evaluated by disabled people themselves and their organizations (French & Swain 2000). Barnes (2004), however, believes that the emancipatory research paradigm has had a demonstrable and significant impact on organizations and researchers doing disability research. Numerous projects on direct payments and personal assistance, for instance, made a significant contribution to the passing of the Community Care (Direct Payment) Act (1996). Barnes is mindful, however, that research is enmeshed within a political and cultural context which may determine how, if at all, it is used. He states (2004:52):

> Research outcomes in themselves cannot bring about meaningful political and social transformation, but they can reinforce and stimulate the demand for change. Thus the main targets for emancipatory research are disabled people and their allies.

To complicate the matter even further, Walmsley & Johnson (2003) use the term 'inclusive research' when talking about research with people with learning disabilities. They argue that inclusive research originates from qualitative research and encompasses some aspects of participatory and emancipatory research. Below are listed the major tenets of inclusive research:

- It must address issues that matter to people with learning disabilities. The research problem must be owned (but not necessarily initiated) by people with learning disabilities.

- It must represent the views and experiences of people with learning disabilities.
- It should further the interests of people with learning disabilities.
- Researchers must 'be on the side' of people with learning disabilities.
- It should be collaborative with people with learning disabilities who should be involved in the research.
- People with learning disabilities should have some control over the process and the outcome of the research.
- People with learning disabilities must be treated with respect by the research community.
- All aspects of the research and the research outcomes should be made accessible to people with learning disabilities.

◆ *Activity 11.6*

THE PLACE OF 'INCLUSIVE' RESEARCH

Walmsley & Johnson (2003) do not believe that emancipatory research can be fully applied when working with people with learning disabilities. Read through the section on emancipatory research again (p. 197) and write a few notes on the possible reasons why Walmsley & Johnson prefer to work within the framework of 'inclusive' research.

Walmsley & Johnson (2003) admit that inclusive research is 'top down' rather than 'bottom up' – that is, it is frequently initiated by the researchers rather than people with learning disabilities themselves. They do not, however, believe that this is necessarily a problem and cite research questions within the social sciences which have emerged from 'silences', such as those concerned with domestic violence and child abuse. They believe that, although people with learning disabilities have an enormous amount of expertise and that those who are less disabled can work as researchers in many ways, it is unrealistic to expect them to fully control the research process that the emancipatory paradigm demands. They go as far as to refer to this expectation as 'unrealistic' and 'oppressive' and state (2003:187):

> to argue that they have the expertise to carry out or control all aspects of research is to go beyond the realms of the rational into a world where the reality of intellectual impairment is wished away and difference is denied.

Walmsley & Johnson (2003) argue further that researchers who work within an inclusive ideology are helping people with learning disabilities to understand their situation, rather than oppressing them, and that without this assistance they may not get beyond telling their stories, however important and empowering that may be. They state that, without allies, research in the area of learning disability may remain '... the untheorized, experienced-based poor relation of its intellectually wealthier cousin in disability studies' (2003:186).

They also defend the position of researchers who work in this way because, although it is likely that they benefit more from the research than people with learning disabilities, their work does not attract funding or status within academic circles and they are frequently marginalized. The power imbalance between the researcher and the researched cannot, they believe, be resolved until society is a more just place for people with learning difficulties.

INVOLVING DISABLED PEOPLE IN RESEARCH

In this section we shall look at some projects with disabled people that involve them and give their perspectives. These projects have been selected to reflect a range of topics and participant groups relevant to physiotherapists and occupational therapists.

Closs (1998) explored the views of children and young people with life-threatening or life-shortening medical conditions. Six young people participated in the study by reflecting on their childhoods, responding to key issues in the literature and criticizing the researchers' drafts. A number of themes were extracted from the data which were considered critical to the quality of the young people's lives, including: the individual's understanding of his or her condition; feelings of sameness/difference; educational experiences and attainments; friendships; family; and experience of the medical and paramedical services and hospital life. In relation to the last of these themes, comments from the young people illustrated some distressing experiences, such as 'If they didn't call it treatment you could call it torture', 'I could write a book about doctors, good, bad and unspeakable', and 'I realised I had nothing on under the sheet. Maybe it was easier for them to put in tubes ... but I felt really embarrassed' (Closs 1998:121). Some enjoyable experiences were also recounted. One participant said 'I don't think you can live for too long in the dumps. I've had lots of laughs, lots of highs' (Closs 1998:116).

Fifty people with aphasia were involved in a study by Parr et al (1997). In-depth interviews were adopted to allow important topics and issues to be raised by the participants, in addition to those on the researchers' agenda. One topic was people's experiences of services. From participants' detailed accounts, attributes of successful services included: availability and accessibility; appropriateness and adequacy; flexibility and responsiveness; integration; reliability and consistency; respectfulness; ability to support communication; and ability to provide relevant and accessible information (Parr et al 1997:66). The experiences of individual participants varied greatly. Madge felt that she had been supported and that the care she had received had been satisfactory. Rebecca's views were, however, very different:

> When you can't communicate they treat you like a kid and that is just so frustrating. A handful of doctors were just awful. You just wanted to say, 'Do you know what this is like?'
>
> (Parr et al 1997:74)

This research is very important because it was the first extensive study of aphasia from the perspective of people with aphasia themselves. It demonstrates that people with impaired language can, under the right conditions, be interviewed and that their views can be used to inform professionals and improve services.

Atkin et al (2000) report on parents' perspectives of the treatment their children with thalassaemia and sickle cell disorder received. Sixty-two interviews with parents were conducted, 21 of which were in languages other than English. Semi-structured interviews were adopted as, '... this approach is particularly recommended for the study of the ways that individuals express their understanding of themselves in the context of their social, cultural and personal circumstances' (Atkin et al 2000:108). Atkin et al (2000) found that the parents faced many problems in having their needs recognized, obtaining necessary information about their child's condition and sources of support, and dealing with poorly co-ordinated services and unsympathetic and poorly informed professionals. One parent explained (Atkin et al 2000:114):

> The medical side should be a bit more informed about the illness so they can inform us about it, but I mean we've come across doctors, nurses ... and they've turned round and said, 'Well I don't know anything about sickle cell.' So straight away, I mean I doubt them straight away. I think, 'Well why are they caring for my child if they don't know anything about it?'

The next example comes from research with people with learning difficulties. Atkinson (1997), along with others, has been developing an

auto/biographical approach that has the capacity to combine the political document with the historical – to reflect the lives which have been
lived, but to see beyond the individuals to a wider view of learning disability. Auto/biography contains many voices and tells stories at different levels.

(Atkinson 1997:22)

Individual life stories were recounted and shared in a group context.
Nine participants with an age range of 57–77 years met on 30 occasions.
One of the themes was 'tales of hospital life' and the following is a short
extract in which Margaret tells her story of running away from a mental handicap hospital (Atkinson 1997:91):

> The sister would keep on at me, saying my work wasn't done
> properly. She was being horrible. I'd scrubbed the ward and she
> said I had to do it over again. I said, 'Well I ain't going to do it over
> again!' I told the doctor. He come round and he wanted to know
> what I was doing on the stairs again. I said, 'I've been told I've got
> to do it again, it wasn't done properly.'

> I planned it with the other girl, we planned it together. She was
> fed up. She was doing the dayroom and dining room, cleaning
> and polishing. Then I was put on it, as well as scrubbing. We
> planned to get into Bedford, walk across the fields.

The following two examples are from therapy research. Martlew (1996),
a physiotherapist, evaluated on-site physiotherapy in a day hospice providing care for patients with terminal illness, using 'client-centred action
research'. She concluded that the learning experience was (1996:564):

> greater because this study was conducted by a practitioner–
> researcher doing her own action research … this study has con-
> firmed the benefit of taking time to listen sensitively – both for the
> professionals, to gain greater insight into patient problems, hope-
> fully leading to more appropriate and therefore effective interven-
> tion; and for patients who feel supported and understood.

Blanche (1996), an occupational therapist, explored the effect of cultural
differences on the delivery of healthcare services through a life story
approach with the mother of a disabled child. She used a 'co-operative
story making' approach which rejects the ideology of 'observed versus
observer' and sees both the interviewer and the informer as building
the story together. She concluded that (1996:274–275):

> clinicians need to acknowledge the client's and their own culture as
> well as the perceptions, expectations, values, and beliefs that are
> inherent in each … Stereotyping persons and treating them as

homogeneous ethnic or racial groups saves time but is not effective. Listening to a client's life story may give us the information we need to place our services within the complexity of his or her life.

Finally we will discuss a more fully developed example of participatory research in that the participants were involved in the decision-making process throughout the research. The project was controlled, conducted and reported, with support, by the Bristol Self-Advocacy Research Group, a group of four people with learning difficulties, and was funded by the National Lottery Fund (Palmer et al 1999). The research involved interviewing other people with learning difficulties about their experiences. The response of the researchers was positive (Palmer et al 1999:34):

> We've all really enjoyed the research visits, meeting new people and making new friends.

> I was looking at my photographs yesterday when I was at home, and all the different places I've been. And I've got the photographs in my photograph album at home. I'm quite proud of what I did. And you feel very important. People say: 'You do do a lot.' They're quite impressed with what I do. I've achieved a lot – too much.

The themes covered in this research were: what is disability?; cutting out all the labels; jobs and work; the staff who support us; transport; and self-advocacy – what does it mean? Under the theme of support, for example, the research participants speak about being forced to be independent (Palmer et al 1999:42):

> Staff people always think that we all want to be more and more independent. This can be wrong, because they expect us to do too many things ourselves. It should be our choice, not theirs.

> If you're married, you've got to give and take. One person does one thing, and people help each other out. It's the same in any house – I don't want staff to keep on forcing me to be independent. How would they feel?

We hope that these examples give an indication of how the principles of participatory and emancipatory research, to a greater or lesser extent, can be applied to research in order to gain a better understanding of issues from the viewpoint of disabled people. Although the examples we have chosen focus largely on disabled people's attitudes and opinions within the sphere of social science research, there is no reason to believe that disabled people cannot be involved in any type of research, although their involvement may bring to the fore different perspectives between disabled people and therapists – not least about what is worth researching.

◆ *Activity* *11.7*

INCLUDING DISABLED PEOPLE IN RESEARCH

Go to the library and select any piece of research that focuses on the lives of disabled people. Look carefully at the methodology and all other aspects of the research, including the formulation of the research question and the dissemination of the findings, and write some notes on how the research could have been more participatory or emancipatory and what the implications of this might be. If possible, compare your notes with a colleague.

CONCLUSION

Research of any kind may seem somewhat removed from the everyday pressures of practising therapists, although most will have had considerable exposure to research ideas and practice during their undergraduate education. Physiotherapists and occupational therapists are, however, in an ideal position to involve disabled people in research. Unlike many health professionals, physiotherapists and occupational therapists frequently spend considerable time with their patients and clients and are in a position to get to know them as people. Sensitive, empowering research can give invaluable insights into patients' and clients' complex experiences of illness, disability and impairment which may, in turn, have the potential to improve therapy practice as well as patient and client satisfaction. Many patients and clients live with disability and impairment on a daily basis and the knowledge and experience they have gained should not be underestimated, however young they may be.

Disabled people have spoken out about the way their perceptions of disability frequently clash with those of health professionals, and non-disabled people in general, and how the neglect of their perspective has created inappropriate and abusive policy and practice. Brothers et al (2002) believe that health professionals need to consult with disabled customers, disabled staff and disability organizations in order to prevent discrimination. With the implementation and strengthening of the Disability Discrimination Act (1995) and the growing philosophy of working with patients and clients in partnership and collaboration, a move towards participatory and emancipatory research in physiotherapy and occupational therapy is long overdue.

We will end this chapter with a question from Mike Oliver (1992:102), who was the first Professor of Disability Studies and a disabled person himself:

> do researchers wish to join with disabled people and use their expertise and skills in their struggles against oppression or do they wish to continue to use these skills and expertise in ways in which disabled people find oppressive?

Disabled people are being empowered by the disabled people's movement. The question is: can research by physiotherapists and occupational therapists be part of that empowerment?

Chapter 12

Reflecting back to reflect forward

In this final chapter we shall attempt to draw together and help you draw together the debates in this book. In doing so we are aware that readers will have differed considerably in their specific purposes, expectations and needs in picking this book up. You will have approached this book in your own way: whether or not you took detailed notes, how many of the activities you responded to and the context in which you read the book, for instance whether or not it was part of a course you were undertaking.

The title of this chapter is an expression of our approach to exploring the implications of disability studies for therapy practice. It is a questioning process addressing how and why structures and processes have developed, to project forward towards possibilities for change. The keys to this approach are in addressing the complexity of issues behind what can seem like 'common sense'. These include:

- prioritizing the voices of disabled people
- introducing the field of disability studies
- exploring the implications of the social model of disability in therapy practice
- acknowledging and critiquing the power relations between people who provide and people who use services
- acknowledging the strengths that you bring to therapy practice
- supporting you in developing your understanding of disability issues and their relevance to therapy practice.

We shall pull all this together under several themes that have developed throughout this book: understanding disability; analysing therapy practice, the possibilities and constraints; developing possibilities for change in realizing effective and good practice; and, ultimately, contributing to full citizenship for disabled people, that is independent living, equality and justice. The chapter is mainly based around activities aimed to help you think of the implications of disability studies for therapy practice.

WHAT IS DISABILITY?

 ### *Activity 12.1*

WHAT DOES DISABILITY MEAN TO YOU?

We return first to the question you were asked in Activity 2.1.

Write down a few words and phrases that, for you, convey the meaning of the word 'disability'.

Compare your responses now with the notes you made for Activity 2.1. How did your thinking develop as you progressed through the book? Why do you think your responses have remained the same or have changed significantly?

As in Chapter 2, we would point out that your responses to this activity will depend on many factors, whether or not reading this book has influenced your thinking. Your experiences in the provision of therapy and your reflections on your experiences may have been significant. Furthermore we are continuously immersed in images and meanings of disability as conveyed through the media. As we write, headline news is the diagnosis of Gordon Brown's child as having cystic fibrosis. Media coverage has been replete with assumptions about disability and particularly the personal responses of parents of disabled children. To give just one further recent example, the headline in *The Sunday Times* (Templeton 2006) read: 'Doctors: Let Us Kill Disabled Babies'. Whatever the ins and outs of the debate within the report are, the tragedy message is writ large in the headline: better dead than disabled. And who says so? It is the 'experts' whose profession is seemingly committed to the preservation of life and health.

At this point, we shall return to the differing standpoints generated by four models of understanding disability and impairment: the medical/individual, the social, the tragedy and the affirmative models. These were introduced in Chapter 2 and have underpinned discussions in the remaining chapters.

Activity 12.2

CONTRASTING MODELS OF DISABILITY

Table 12.1 presents questions for you to complete. Try to fill in each cell illustrating the different possible answers from each of the models. We hope you will find some cells quite easy, such as answering 'What is the problem?' Others may be rather more difficult, but are worth thinking through.

Table 12.1

	Individual/ medical model	Social model	Tragedy model	Affirmative model
What is the problem?				
In what ways do individuals need to change?				
In what ways do services need to change?				
What are the politics of disability?				
What are the visions of the future?				

Our version of the completed table is included as an Appendix at the end of the chapter. It is based on Oliver's (1996) original idea for contrasting the medical and social models of disability. Differentiating and characterizing different ways of thinking about and responding to disability and impairment lie at the heart of this exercise. Standing back from the exercise, it is important to recognize that we are characterizing viewpoints. Within each there is a diversity of opinions. The charity model, medical model, administrative model and tragedy model, for instance, can all be thought of as differing versions of the individual model. The affirmative model is simply a different version of the social model. Furthermore, models of disability are continually evolving and are dynamic and changing rather than static and agreed universally. Perhaps most controversial is what can be seen as a sharp and absolute division of views, that is the individual/medical model versus the social model, and the tragedy model versus the affirmative model. It can be argued that these reflect a continuum of thinking rather than being dichotomies. Nevertheless, this is not simply an academic exercise. The implications for analysing and developing therapy practice are far-reaching.

REFLECTING ON THERAPY PRACTICE

Our second theme has been critical reflection on policy, practice and provision. This began in Chapter 1, not just by the raising of questions and more questions, but by the questioning of questions.

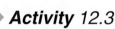

Activity 12.3

WHAT IS GOOD PRACTICE?

We asked the same question in Activity 1.1 as a starting point for studying disability and the implications for therapy. At that stage, you may remember, we used the question to raise other questions such as who decides what is good practice and on what basis. Though we believe this is a good approach to studying disability issues, you may have found it rather frustrating – to be always questioning and not finding answers. We return now to that first question, but as informed by your studies of disability issues. So take a little time to consider the following question. In doing so you may find it useful to look through any notes you have made for activities throughout the book.

What is good practice as informed by disability studies?

As we have emphasized, the implications of disability studies, the social and affirmative models, do not translate in any mechanical or 'cookbook' way into recipes for therapy policy, practice and provision. Nor do they, in any simple way, negate the importance of effective therapy practice and medical interventions for disabled people. Nevertheless, as we hope you have seen, the whole arena of disability studies raises farreaching questions. It challenges the status quo, and, more positively, generates principles through which good practice can be informed.

- The first is the recognition and mobilizing of disabled people's, and their close associates', established knowledge, capabilities, aspirations and resources in order to combat stress and discrimination and promote resilience. This 'empowerment approach' focuses on the strengthening and facilitation of individual interpersonal and political power among disabled service users.

- The voices of disabled people in controlling policy, practice and provision are paramount within the social model of disability. Within this the notion and imperative of independent living has, in more recent years, played a crucial role.

- As explored in Chapter 10, the implications for therapy practice, policy and provision incorporate social and cultural considerations, beyond disability issues. Disability issues cannot be addressed without the accommodation of the needs, values, goals and systems relating to sexism, ageism, sexual preference and the discrimination faced by ethnic minority communities.

- Disability studies engages with the critique of existing therapy policy, practice and provision. A recurring theme in previous chapters, and in the documented experiences of disabled people, has been professional practice and provision of services as frequently part of 'the problem' rather than 'the solution'.

- Critical reflection casts light on the cultural and experiential background (sometimes derogatively called 'baggage') that you bring, as a therapist, to therapy practice with disabled people. The individual model, in its various guises, is deeply ingrained within our culture and society. This builds, sometimes insidiously, through the messages of tragedy, incapability, dependency and abnormality rampant within the media. More direct, in terms of therapy practice, is the dominance of the medical model of disability not only as the foundation for intervention but also as integral to the culture of organizations. In this context the social and affirmative models generate critical reflection. The meaning and value of the clients' viewpoints are prioritized – what they bring to therapy, the meaning of therapy for clients and their evaluation of therapy in relation to their lives. Critical reflection can be creative, too, in terms of support for clients in control over decision making within the therapy process.

- Finally, education is clearly important – and in particular the incorporation of disability studies in professional education. Sinclair (2005:xiv), recognizing the radical implications of such a wide perspective for practice, suggests that:

> Occupational therapists must develop their roles as agents of social change, taking the profession to a new level that makes a

difference to entire communities as well as to the individuals we treat and encourage. To enable them to become effective agents of change the way in which occupational therapists are educated must come under sweeping review.

REFLECTING FORWARD

Our third theme has been perhaps the most challenging. It takes therapists beyond the minutiae of daily therapy practice towards engaging with disability as a political issue. Connecting with disability studies and disability issues can take therapists beyond clinical settings, beyond assessment and interventions with individuals, to address their role in social change. This is not to deny the importance of the medical expertise of therapists or effective medical intervention. It is the engagement of therapists' expertise, in support of and partnership with disabled people, in the creation of a society in which all disabled people are able to participate as equal citizens.

Activity 12.4

WHAT ARE THE POSSIBILITIES FOR SOCIAL CHANGE?

In a chapter entitled 'Disability, Struggle and the Politics of Hope', Len Barton (2001:10) writes:

... disabled people are demanding changes. They are not arguing for sameness, or to become as normal as possible, nor are they seeking an independence without assistance. Their vision is of a world in which discrimination and injustice are removed. They are desirous of the establishment of alternative definitions and perceptions based on a dignified view of difference. The struggle for inclusion is thus disturbing, demanding and developmental. It involves the experience of exercising choices and rights ...

In this final activity, let us join Len Barton and disabled people in thinking about this vision for justice and the removal of discrimination. He writes about the politics of hope. Drawing on your studies of disability issues what do you see as the main sources of hope in realizing this vision? More research? Better services? More resources? Such 'crystal ball' questions are not, of course, easy to answer.

With some trepidation we would suggest the following are important sources of hope at present.

1. The collective struggle for social change by disabled people

The disabled people's movement was a key factor in the emergence of disability studies as an academic discipline in its own right. The collective voice of disabled people remains for many, including ourselves, the vanguard of social change for disabled people. The British Council of Disabled People (recently renamed the United Kingdom's Disabled People's Council) is the main umbrella organization of disabled people. The following short extract from their manifesto (2005) refers to the provision of services and support:

> BCODP calls for local authorities and health services to work together where needed to give disabled people the chance to be responsible for working out and saying what their own needs are. Services should fit around the needs of individual disabled people and give them support to make decisions and to lead full and active lives.

For disabled people the vision of social change has increasingly come under the banner of independent living. The Disability Rights Commission (2002:5) has defined independent living as disabled people '... having the same choice, control and freedom as any other citizen – at home, at work, and as members of the community. This does not necessarily mean disabled people "doing everything for themselves", but it does mean that any practical assistance people need should be based on their own choices and aspirations'. The realization of this ideal includes equal access to mainstream education (schools, colleges and universities), paid employment, transport, 'public' buildings, housing, leisure and health and social care services. This idea of independent living, as defined by disabled people themselves, is founded on four basic assumptions.

1. All human beings are of equal worth, regardless of the nature, complexity or severity of their impairments.

2. Everyone, regardless of the nature, complexity or severity of their impairments, has the capacity to make choices in controlling their lifestyles and should be supported in making such choices.

3. Disabled people have the right to exercise control over their lives.

4. Disabled people have the right to participate fully in all areas, economic, political and cultural of mainstream community living on an equal basis with their non-disabled peers.

The National Centre for Independent Living (2006:35) states:

> The independent living movement has identified peer support and participation as key to empowerment, where disabled people share experience and expertise – formally or informally via user networks or meetings and peer mentoring. Independent living training for users is also part of the equation. Independent living is about a shift of power from professionals to disabled people – and in this respect, disabled people's involvement at all levels of a direct payments support organisation is an essential ingredient of success.

2. Anti-discrimination legislation and national policy

The creation of participative citizenship for disabled people will involve the strengthening and enforcement of legislation and procedures to ensure that disability and independent living issues are fully integrated into policy making at all levels: international, national, regional and local. This includes the enactment of binding and intractable anti-discrimination legislation with effective enforcement and compliance requirements.

The imperative of independent living is being recognized within national policy. In the report from the Prime Minister's Strategy Unit (2005:7), independent living is the first strategy specified:

> ... helping disabled people to achieve independent living by moving progressively to individual budgets for disabled people, drawing together the services to which they are entitled and giving them greater choice over the mix of support they receive in the form of cash and/or direct provision of services. In the shorter term, measures should also be taken to improve the advice services available to disabled people and to address existing problems with suitable housing and transport.

Furthermore the Independent Living Bill has recently been through its second reading. The principles of the bill are:

- support, freedom, choice and control by disabled people
- the right to self-determination
- action to address discrimination against marginalized groups, including older disabled people and disabled people from black and minority ethnic communities
- protection of dignity and family life
- protection of the health of carers.

Mainstreaming is also a key concept. The mainstreaming of disability issues within policy agendas addresses the marginalization of the needs and rights of disabled people and their treatment as a 'special' case. This presents fundamental challenges to policy making in realizing the prerogatives of flexibility, the expertise of disabled people and the recognition that 'one size does not fit all'. It requires the breaking down of the physical, social, communication and economic barriers that prevent disabled people from exercising their rights and participating in policy making. Some of these barriers are embedded in the local circumstances in which disabled people live their lives, experienced as lack of choice and control in style and quality of life. Some are embedded in the processes of policy making and the practicalities of enforcement mechanisms in achieving the needs and rights of disabled people.

3. Control of support and services

Centres for Independent Living have provided the means for control of services by disabled people and the blueprint for changing relationships between service providers and service users. The influence on national policy is clear in the following recommendation within the report from The Prime Minister's Strategy Unit (2005:90):

> By 2010, each locality (defined as that area covered by a council with social services responsibilities) should have a user-led organisation modeled on existing CILs.

4. Broad social, cultural and economic change

All visions for a better society are constructed in particular social and historical contexts. Looking at our ever more rapidly changing society it is difficult to identify forces of change that indisputably feed a politics of hope for disabled people. Nevertheless, the democratic and participatory possibilities afforded by the Internet and other technological developments are potentially significant. These developments have opened up opportunities for dialogic, or participative, democracy rather than representative democracy. The Internet allows for greater diversity or plurality of voices to be heard and has the potential to be profoundly democratizing. The Internet generates truly global electronic communities, and new forms of participation and community. Bulletin boards, websites and email engender democratic possibilities and their use by disabled peoples' organizations testify to their utility in democratic processes. The possibilities of an international perspective on disability, then, can be realized. An international perspective on disability challenges the global structures that lock millions of disabled people into poverty and silence. The danger is the possibility of the further marginalization of 'the unconnected', the disabled people who are the poorest of the poor for whom survival is the political perspective, and for whom sophisticated technology is not available. It is also the case that new technologies are developed within disabling societies and are not available to many disabled people unless adaptations are developed and implemented.

5. And ...

We have purposefully ended on a positive note of hope. Overall, paramount to the vision of a society inclusive of disabled people is the emerging voices of disabled people in controlling decision-making processes across policy and research that shapes their day-to-day lifestyles, opportunities and choices. It is an ongoing struggle for a truly equitable and inclusive society with justice and full participative citizenship for all. We hope this book has supported you in becoming an active agent in social change, and in acknowledging, supporting and promoting the voices of disabled people and their continuing struggle for a society fit for all.

APPENDIX: CONTRASTING MODELS OF DISABILITY

	Individual/ medical model	Social model	Tragedy model	Affirmative model
What is the problem?	The individual; the individual's impairment	The barriers to participation in a disabling society	The tragedy of suffering from an impairment and living a disabled lifestyle	Presumptions that people with impairments see themselves and their lives as tragic
In what ways do individuals need to change?	To be more normal	To transform consciousness: the society rather than the individual causes disablement	To accept and come to terms with the tragedy	To affirm a non-tragedy, positive identity
In what ways do services need to change?	By improving existing services	By the control of different services by disabled people	By disabled people understanding that they are privileged to receive existing services and benefits	By disabled people controlling services that affirm positive identity and lifestyle from the standpoint of disabled people
What are the politics of disability?	Empowerment as a gift from those with power	Self-empowerment as a struggle of the powerless	Beyond the scope and lives of those suffering tragedy	Individual and collective affirmation of self, lifestyles, quality of life by disabled people
What are the visions of the future?	A normal society with effective care and cure services	Full participation Full citizenship Equal opportunities Equal rights	The elimination of tragedy: the elimination of or removal from society of disabled people	Celebration of differences Recognition of disability culture and pride

References

Abberley P 1992 Counting us out: a discussion of the OPCS disability surveys. Disability Handicap and Society 7:139–155

Abberley P 1995 Disabling ideology in health and welfare – the case of occupational therapy. Disability and Society 10(2):221–232

Abbott P, Meerabeau L 1998 Professionals, professionalisation and the caring professions. In: Abbott P, Meerabeau L (eds) The sociology of the caring professions. UCL Press, London, p. 1–19

Ahmad WIU, Atkin K (eds) 1998 Race and community care. Open University Press, Buckingham

Andrews J 2005 The rise of the asylum in Britain. In: Brunton D (ed.) Medicine transformed: health disease and society in Europe, 1800–1930. Manchester University Press, Manchester, p. 298–330

Anionwu E 1996 Ethnic origin of sickle cell and thalassaemia counsellors. In: Kelleher D, Hillier S (eds) Researching cultural differences in health. Routledge, London, p. 160–189

Anionwu E, Atkin K 2001 The politics of sickle cell and thalassaemia. Open University Press, Buckingham

Ashton H, Rodgers J 2005 A health promoting empowerment approach to diabetes nursing. In: Scriven A (ed.) Health promoting practice: the contribution of nurses and allied health professionals. Palgrave Macmillan, Houndmills, p. 45–56

Atkin K, Ahmad WIU, Anionwu E 2000 Service support to families caring for a child with a sickle cell disorder or beta thalassaemia major: parents' perspectives. In: Ahmad WIU (ed.) Ethnicity disability and chronic illness. Open University Press, Buckingham, p. 103–122

Atkin K, French S, Vernon A 2004 Health care for people from ethnic minority groups. In: French S, Sim J (eds) Physiotherapy: a psychosocial approach, 3rd edn. Butterworth-Heinemann, Oxford, p. 83–94

Atkinson D 1997 An auto/biographical approach to learning disability research. Ashgate, Aldershot

Atkinson D, Jackson M, Walmsley J 1997 Forgotton lives: exploring the history of learning disability. British Institute of Learning Disability, Kidderminster

Ballard K, McDonald T 1999 Disability inclusion and exclusion: some insider accounts and interpretations. In: Ballard K (ed.) Inclusive education: international voices on disability and justice. Falmar, London, p. 97–115

Barclay J 1994 In good hands: the history of the Chartered Society of Physiotherapy. The Chartered Society of Physiotherapy, London

Barnes C 1991 Disabled people in Britain and discrimination: a case for anti-discrimination legislation. Hurst/University of Calgary Press, London

Barnes C 1992 Disabling imagery and the media. The British Council of Organisations of Disabled People, Derby

Barnes C 2001 Emancipatory disability research: project or process? Public lecture for the Strathclyde Centre for Disability Research, University of Glasgow. Online. Available: http://www.leeds.ac.uk/disability-studies/archiveuk/ Accessed April 2007

Barnes C 2004 Reflections on doing emancipatory disability research. In: Swain J, French S, Barnes C, Thomas C (eds) Disabling barriers – enabling environments, 2nd edn. Sage, London, p. 47–53

Barnes M, Bowl R 2001 Taking over the asylum: empowerment and mental health. Palgrave, Houndmills

Barnes C, Mercer G 1997 Doing disability research. The Disability Press, Leeds

Barnes C, Mercer G (eds) 2004 Implementing the social model of disability: theory and research. The Disability Press, Leeds

Barnes C, Mercer G 2006 Independent futures: creating user-led disability services in a disabling society. Policy Press, Bristol

Barnes M, Harrison S, Mort M, Shardlow P 1999a Unequal partners: user group and community care. Policy Press, Bristol

Barnes C, Mercer G, Shakespeare T 1999b Exploring disability: a sociological introduction. Polity Press, Cambridge

Barton L 1998 Developing an emancipatory research agenda: possibilities and dilemmas. In: Clough P, Barton L (eds) Articulating with difficulty: research voices in inclusive education. Paul Chapman, London, p. 29–39

Barton L 2001 Disability struggle and the politics of hope. In: Barton L (ed.) Disability politics and the struggle for change. David Fulton, London, p. 1–23

Barton L 2004 The disability movement: some observations. In: Swain J, French S, Barnes C, Thomas C (eds) Disabling barriers – enabling environments, 2nd edn. Sage, London, p. 285–290

Basnett I 2001 Health care professionals and their attitudes towards and decisions affecting disabled people. In: Albrecht G, Seelman KD, Bury M (eds) Handbook of disability studies. Sage, London, p. 450–467

Battye L 1966 The Chatterley syndrome. In: Hunt P (ed.) Stigma: the experience of disability. Chapman, London, p. 3–18

BBC Radio 4 2002 Archive hour: Thalidomide: 40 Years. BBC Radio 4, June 1

Beeton K in press An exploration of the quality of life of adults with haemophilia. In French S, Swain J (eds) Disability on equal terms: understanding and valuing difference. Sage, London

Begum N 1994 Snow White. In: Keith L (ed.) Mustn't grumble: writing by disabled women. The Women's Press, London

Begum N 1996 Doctor doctor…: disabled women's experiences of general practitioners. In: Morris J (ed.) Encounters with strangers: feminism and disability. The Women's Press, London, p. 168–193

Belle Brown J, Stewart M, Wayne Weston W et al 2003 Introduction. In: Stewart M, Belle Brown J, Wayne Weston W et al (eds) Patient-centred medicine: transforming the clinical method, 2nd edn. Sage, London, p. 3–16

Benzeval M, Judge K, Whitehead M 1995a Introduction. In: Benzeval M, Judge K, Whitehead M (eds) Tackling inequalities in health: an agenda for action. Kings Fund, London, p. 1–9

Benzeval M, Judge K, Whitehead M 1995b The role of the NHS. In: Benzeval M, Judge K, Whitehead M (eds) Tackling inequalities in health: an agenda for action. Kings Fund, London, p. 96–121

Beresford P 2006 Empowerment and emancipation. In: Albrecht GL (ed.) Encyclopedia of disability, Vol 2. Sage, Thousand Oaks, p. 593–600

Beresford P, Campbell J 1994 Disabled people, service users, user involvement and representation. Disability Handicap and Society 93:315–325

Beresford P, Croft S 2000 User participation. In: Davies M (ed.) The Blackwell encyclopaedia of social work. Blackwell, Oxford, p. 355–357

Beresford P, Croft S, Evans C et al 1997 Quality in personal social services: the developing role of user involvement in the UK. In: Evans A, Haverinen K, Leichsering K et al (eds) Developing quality in personal social services. Ashgate, Aldershot, p. 63–80

Bewley C, Glendinning C 1994 Involving disabled people in community care planning. Joseph Rowntree Foundation, York

Bignall T, Butt J 2000 Between ambition and achievement: young Black disabled people's views and experiences of independence and independent living. Policy Press, Bristol

Blakemore K 1998 Social policy: an introduction. Open University Press, Buckingham

Blanche E 1996 Alma: coping with culture poverty and disability. American Journal of Occupational Therapy 50:265–274

Boazman S 1999 Inside aphasia. In: Corker M, French S (eds) Disability discourse. Open University Press, Buckingham, p. 15–20

Borsay A 2005 Disability and social policy in Britain since 1750. Palgrave, Basingstoke

Bourke J 1996 Dismembering the male: men's bodies, Britain and the great war. Reaktion Books, London

Braye S 2000 Participation and involvement in social care: an overview. In: Kemshall H, Littlechild R (eds) User involvement and participation in social care. Jessica Kingsley, London, p. 9–28

Braye S, Preston-Shoot M 1995 Empowering practice in social care. Open University Press, Buckingham

Brechin A 1993 Sharing. In: Shakespeare P, Atkinson D, French S (eds) Reflecting on research practice: issues in health and social care. Open University Press, Buckingham, p. 70–82

Brechin A 2000 Introducing critical practice. In: Brechin A, Brown H, Eby MA (eds) Critical practice in health and social care. Sage, London, p. 25–47

Brechin A, Brown H, Eby MA (eds) 2000 Critical practice in health and social care. Sage, London

Brigham L, Atkinson D, Jackson M et al 2000 Crossing boundaries: change and continuity in the history of learning disability. British Institute of Learning Disabilities, Kidderminster

British Council of Disabled People 2003 The social model of disability and emancipatory disability research – briefing document. British Council of Disabled People, Derby. Online. Available: http://www.bcodp.org.uk Accessed April 2007

British Council of Disabled People 2005 The voice of disabled people still fighting for full rights: 2005 manifesto. British Council of Disabled People, Derby. Online. Available: http://www.bcodp.org.uk Accessed April 2007

Brothers M, Scullion P, Eathorne V 2002 Rights of access to services for disabled people. British Journal of Therapy and Rehabilitation 9:232–236

Brown H 2000 Challenges from service users. In: Brechin A, Brown H, Eby MA (eds) Critical practice in health and social care. Sage, London, p. 96–116

Brunton D 2004 The emergence of a modern profession. In: Brunton D (ed.) Medicine transformed: health disability and society in Europe 1800–1930. Cambridge University Press, Cambridge, p. 119–150

Burchardt T 2000 Enduring economic exclusion: disabled people, income and work. Joseph Rowntree Foundation, York

Burchardt T 2005 The education and employment of disabled young people: frustrated ambition. Joseph Rowntree Foundation, York

Burnard P 1992 Counselling: a guide to practice in nursing. Butterworth-Heinemann, Oxford

Butler J, Calnan M 1999 Health and health policy. In: Baldock J, Manning N, Miller S et al (eds) Social policy. Oxford University Press, Oxford, p. 310–343

Butt J, Mirza K 1996 Social care and Black communities. Race Equality Unit, London

Byron M, Howell C, Bradley P et al 2005 Different differences: disability equality teaching in healthcare education. University of Bristol, Bristol

Campbell J, Oliver M 1996 Disability politics: understanding our past, changing our future. Routledge, London

Cant S 2005 Understanding why people use complementary and alternative medicine. In: Heller T, Lee-Treweek G, Katz J et al (eds) Perspectives on complementary and alternative medicine. Routledge, London, p. 173–204

Carmichael A 2004 The social model, the emancipatory paradigm and user involvement. In: Barnes C, Mercer G (eds) Implementing the social model of disability: theory and research. The Disability Press, Leeds, p. 191–207

Carnwell R, Buchanan J (eds) 2005 Effective practice in health and social care: a partnership approach. Open University Press, Buckingham

Carr S 2004 Has service user involvement made a difference to social care services? Social Care Institute for Excellence, London

Chafetz ME 1996 The tyranny of experts. Madison Books, London

Chambers R 1997 Whose reality counts: putting the first last. Intermediate Technology Publications, London

Charlton J 2000 Nothing about us without us: disability oppression and empowerment. University of California Press, Berkeley

Chartered Society of Physiotherapy 2002 Rules of professional conduct, 2nd edn. Chartered Society of Physiotherapy, London

Clark L 2002 Liverpool Central Primary Care Trust accessible health information: project report. Online. Available: http://www.leeds.ac.uk/disability-studies Accessed April 2007

Clegg J 2006 Understanding intellectually disabled clients in clinical psychology. In: Goodley D, Lawthom R (eds) Disability and psychology: critical introductions and reflections. Palgrave, Houndmills, p. 123–140

Closs A 1998 Quality of life of children and young people with serious medical conditions. In: Robinson C, Stalker K (eds) Growing up with disability. Jessica Kingsley, London, p. 111–128

Cohen B 2005 Inter-agency collaboration in context: the joining-up agenda. In: Glaister A, Glaister B (eds) Inter-agency collaboration: providing for children. Dundee Academic Press, Edinburgh, p. 1–12

Coleman V 1988 The health scandal: your health in crisis. Sidgwick and Jackson, London

Conrad F, Schneider J 1980 Deviance and medicalisation: from deviance to badness. CV Mosby, St Louis

Cooter R 2004 Medicine in war. In: Brunton D (ed.) Medicine transformed: health disease and society in Europe 1800–1830. Manchester University Press, Manchester, p. 331–363

Corker M 1996 Deaf transitions: images and origins of deaf families, deaf communities and deaf identities. Jessica Kingsley, London

Cornwell A, Jewkes R 1995 What is participatory research? Social Science and Medicine 41:1667–1676

Crow L 1996 Including all of our lives: renewing the social model of disability. In: Morris J (ed.) Encounters with strangers: feminism and disability. The Women's Press, London, p. 206–226

Cunningham CC, Davis H 1985 Working with parents: frameworks for collaboration. Open University Press, Buckingham

Dale N 1996 Working with families of children with special needs: partnership and practice. Routledge, London

D'amour D, Ferrada-Videla M, San Martin Rodriguez L, Beaulieu MD 2005 The conceptual basis for interprofessional collaboration: core concepts and theoretical frameworks. Journal of Interprofessional Care 1:116–131

Davey B 1999 Solving economic, social and environmental problems together: an empowerment strategy for losers. In: Barnes M, Warren L (eds) Paths to empowerment. Policy Press, Bristol, p. 37–50

Davies C 1992 Life times: a mutual biography of disabled people. Understanding Disability Educational Trust, Farnham

Davies C 1998 The cloak of professionalism. In: Allott M, Robb M (eds) Understanding health and social care: an introductory reader. Sage, London, p. 290–297

Davis K 1999 The disabled people's movement: putting the power in empowerment. In: Barnes M, Warren L (eds) Paths to empowerment. Policy Press, Bristol, p. 15–24

Davis JM 2004 Disability and childhood: deconstructing the stereotypes. In Swain J, French S, Barnes C, Thomas C (eds) Disabling barriers – enabling environments, 2nd edn. Sage, London, p. 142–148

Dawson C 2000 Independent successes: implementing direct payments. Joseph Rowntree Foundation, York

Department of Health 1989a Caring for people: community care in the next decade and beyond. HMSO, London

Department of Health 1989b Working for patients. HMSO, London

Department of Health 1991 Managers and practitioners: guide to care management and assessment. HMSO, London

Department of Health 1999 Saving lives: our healthier nation. HMSO, London

Department of Health 2000 The health and social care bill. HMSO, London

Department of Health 2001 The national health inequalities targets. Department of Health, London

Department of Health, Department of the Environment 1992 Housing and community care. HMSO, London

Department of Health, Social Services Inspectorate, Scottish Office Social Work Services Group 1991 Care management and assessment: summary of practice guidance. HMSO/Scottish Office Social Work Services Group, London

de Renzi S 2004 Policies of health: diseases, poverty and hospitals. In: Elmer P (ed.) The healing arts: health disease and society in Europe, 1500–1800. Manchester University Press, Manchester, p. 136–165

Dewey J 1933 How do we think: a restatement of the relation of reflective thinking to the education process. Henry Regnery, Chicago

Disability Rights Commission 2002 Policy statement on social care and independent living. Disability Rights Commission, London

Disability Rights Commission 2005 Independent living briefing – Queen's speech debates. Disability Rights Commission, London

Dominelli L 1997 Anti-racist social work, 2nd edn. Macmillan Press, Houndsmill

Dominelli L 2002 Anti-oppressive social work: theory and practice. Palgrave, Houndmills

Douglas J, Komaromy C, Robb M 2004 Diversity and difference. Communication Unit 6 K205. The Open University, Milton Keynes

Doyal L 1995 What makes women sick: gender and the political economy of health. Macmillan, London

Doyal L 1998 The new obstetrics: science or social control? In: Allott M, Robb M (eds) Understanding health and social care: an introductory reader. Sage, London, p. 123–129

Drake R F 1996 Understanding disability policies. Macmillan, London

Duchan JF 2001 Learning leveling and leveling learning. Graduation speech, Department of Communicative Disorders and Sciences, University of Buffalo, New York. Online. Available: http://www.acsu.buffalo.edu/~duchan/leveling.html Accessed April 2007

Dunton WR 1957 History of occupational therapy. In: Dunton WR, Licht S (eds) Occupational therapy: principles and practice, 2nd edn. Charles C Thomas, Springfield, p. 2–13

Engel GL 1977 The need for a new medical model: a challenge for biomedicine. Science 196:129–126

Esmond D, Gordon K, McCaskie K et al 1998 More scope for fair housing. Scope, London

Evans SE 2004 Forgotten crimes: the holocaust and people with disabilities. Ivan R Dee, Chicago

Ewles L, Simmett I 2003 Promoting health: a practical guide, 5th edn. Baillière Tindall, London

Farrell C 2004 Patient and public involvement in health: the evidence for policy implementation. Department of Health, London

Finkelstein V 1972 The psychology of disability. University of Leeds, Leeds. Online. Available: http://www.leeds.ac.uk/disability-studies/archiveuk/index.html Accessed April 2007

Finkelstein V 1980 Attitudes and disabled people: issues for discussion. Rehabilitation Fund, New York

Finkelstein V 1990 A tale of two cities. Therapy Weekly 16(34):6–7

Finkelstein V 1991 Disability: an administrative challenge? The health and welfare heritage. In: Oliver M (ed.) Social work: disabled people and disabling environments. Jessica Kingsley, London, p. 19–39

Finkelstein V 2004 Modernising services. In: Swain J, French S, Barnes C, Thomas C (eds) Disabling barriers – enabling environments, 2nd edn. Sage, London, p. 206–211

Finkelstein V, Stuart O 1996 Developing new services. In: Hales G (ed.) Beyond disability: towards an enabling society. Sage, London, p. 170–187

Finlay L 2000a The challenge of working in teams. In: Brechin A, Brown H, Eby MA (eds) Critical practice in health and social care. Sage, London, p. 164–185

Finlay L 2000b The challenge of professionalism. In: Brechin A, Brown H, Eby MA (eds) Critical practice in health and social care. Sage, London, p. 141–163

Fitzpatrick M 2001 The tyranny of health: doctors and the regulation of lifestyle. Routledge, London

Fowler HW, Fowler FG (eds) (Revised by McIntosh E) 1964 The concise Oxford dictionary of current English. The Clarendon Press, Oxford

Fox J, Benzeval M 1995 Perspectives on social variations on health. In: Benzeval M, Judge K, Whitehead M (eds) Tackling inequalities in health: an agenda for action. Kings Fund, London, p. 10–21

Freidson E 1970 Profession of medicine: a study of the sociology of applied knowledge. Harper and Row, New York

French S 1986 Handicapped people in the health and caring professions: attitudes, practices and experiences. Unpublished MSc Dissertation, South Bank Polytechnic, London

French S 1987 Attitudes of physiotherapists to the recruitment of disabled and handicapped people into the physiotherapy professions. Physiotherapy 73(7):363–367

French S 1988 Experiences of disabled health and caring professionals. Sociology of Health and Illness 10(2):169–188

French S 1990 The advantages of visual impairment: some physiotherapists' views. New Beacon 74(872):1–6

French S 1994a The disabled role. In: French S (ed.) On equal terms: working with disabled people. Butterworth-Heinemann, Oxford, p. 47–60

French S 1994b Disabled people and professional practice. In: French S (ed.) On equal terms: working with disabled people. Butterworth-Heinemann, Oxford, p. 103–118

French S 1996a Simulation exercises in disability awareness training: a critique. In: Hales G (ed.) Beyond disability: towards an enabling society. Sage, London, p. 114–123

French S 1996b Out of sight out of mind: the experience and effect of a special residential school. In: Morris J (ed.) Encounters with strangers: feminism and disability. The Women's Press, London, p. 17–47

French S 1996c The attitudes of health professionals towards disabled people. In Hales G (ed.) Beyond disability: towards an enabling environment. Sage, London, p. 161–182

French S 1999 Multidisciplinary teams. In: Swain J, French S (eds) Therapy and learning difficulties: advocacy, participation and partnership. Butterworth-Heinemann, Oxford, p. 261–267

French S 2001 Disabled people and employment: a study of the working lives of visually impaired physiotherapists. Ashgate, Aldershot

French S 2004 Enabling relationships in therapy practice In: Swain J, Clark J, Parry K et al Enabling relationships in health and social care: a guide for therapists. Butterworth-Heinemann, Oxford, p. 95–108

French S, Sim J (eds) 2004 Physiotherapy: a psychosocial approach, 3rd edn. Butterworth-Heinemann, Oxford

French S, Swain J 2000 Good intentions: reflecting on researching the lives and experiences of visually disabled people. Annual Review of Critical Psychology 2:35–54

French S, Swain J 2001 The relationship between disabled people and health and welfare professionals. In: Albrecht G, Seelman KD, Bury M (eds) Handbook of disability studies. Sage, London, p. 734–753

French S, Swain J 2004 Controlling inclusion in education: young disabled people's perspectives. In: Swain J, French S, Barnes C, Thomas C (eds) Disabling barriers – enabling environments, 2nd edn. Sage, London, p. 169–175

French S, Swain J 2005 Disability and communication: listening is not enough. In: Robb M, Barrett S, Komaromy C et al (eds) Communication relationships and care: a reader. Routledge, London, p. 120–134

French S, Swain J 2006 Housing: the users' perspectives. In: Clutton S, Grisbrooke J, Pengelly S (eds) Occupational therapy in housing: building on firm foundations. Whurr, Chichester, p. 64–82

French S, Swain J in press User involvement in services for disabled people. In: Jones R, Jenkins F (eds) Management, leadership and development in the allied health professions: an introduction. Radcliffe, Oxford

French S, Vernon A 1997 Health care for people from ethnic minority groups. In: French S (ed.) Physiotherapy: a psychosocial approach, 2nd edn. Butterworth-Heinemann, Oxford, p. 59–72

French S, Gillman M, Swain J 1997 Working with visually disabled people: bridging theory and practice. Venture Press, Birmingham

French S, Reynolds F, Swain J 2001 Practical research: a guide for therapists, 2nd edn. Butterworth-Heinemann, Oxford

French S, Swain J, Atkinson D, Moore M 2006 An oral history of the education of visually impaired people: telling stories for inclusive futures. Edwin Mellen Press, Lampeter

Frontera WR 2006 Medicine. In: Albrecht G (ed.) Encyclopedia of disability, Vol 3. Sage, Thousand Oaks, p. 1067–1074

Fulcher J, Scott J 1999 Sociology. Oxford University Press, Oxford

Ghaye T 2000 Empowerment through reflection: is this a case of the Emperor's new clothes? In: Ghaye T, Gillespie D, Lillyman S (eds) Empowerment through reflection: the narratives of healthcare professionals. Quay Books, Wiltshire

Ghaye T, Lillyman S 2000 Reflection: principles and practice for healthcare professionals. Quay Books, Wiltshire

Gibbs D 2004 Social model services: an oxymoron? In: Barnes C, Mercer G (eds) Disability policy and practice: applying the social model. The Disability Press, Leeds, p. 144–159

Giddens A 2006 Sociology, 5th edn. Polity Press, Cambridge

Gillespie-Sells K, Campbell J 1991 Disability equality training: trainers guide. Central Council for Education and Training in Social Work, London

Goffman E 1963 Stigma: notes on the management of spoiled identity. Prentice-Hall, Englewood Cliffs, New Jersey

Gomm R 1993 Issues of power in health and welfare. In: Walmsley J, Reynolds J, Shakespeare P et al (eds) Health, welfare and practice: reflecting on roles and relationships. Sage, London, p. 131–138

Gough I 1998 What are human needs? In: Franklin J (ed.) Social policy and social justice. Polity Press, Cambridge, p. 50–56

Gould N 1996 Introduction: social work education and the 'crisis of the professions'. In: Gould N, Taylor I (eds) Reflective learning for social work. Arena, Aldershot, p. 1–10

Green V 2005 I see your voice: practicalities, problems and possible solutions for deaf students accessing learning within a health profession course, with specific reference to physiotherapy. Online. Available: http://www.health.heacademy. ac.uk/publications/studentessay/veritygreen/ Accessed April 2007

Hafferty FW 2006 Professions. In: Albrecht GL (ed) Encyclopedia of disability, Vol 3. Sage, Thousand Oaks, p. 1296–1299

Ham C 1999 Health policy in Britain, 4th edn. Palgrave, Basingstoke

Hasler F 2006 Holding the dream: direct payments and independent living. In: Leece J, Bornat J (eds) Developments in direct payments. Polity Press, Bristol, p. 285–292

Heaton M 1998 Listen, you might hear something. Outlook, June 15:12

Heller T 2005 Integration of CAM with mainstream services. In: Heller T, Lee-Treweek G, Katz J et al (eds) Perspectives on complementary and alternative medicine. Routledge, London, p. 379–407

Helman CG 2000 Culture, health and illness: an introduction for health professionals, 4th edn. Butterworth-Heinemann, Oxford

Heywood F 2006 The assessment process. In: Clutton S, Grisbrooke J, Pengelly S (eds) Occupational therapy in housing: building on firm foundations. Whurr, London, p. 21–42

Holliday Wiley L 1999 Pretending to be normal: living with Asperger's syndrome. Jessica Kingsley, London

Homan R 1991 The ethics of social research. Longman, London

Hughes B 2002 Disability and the body. In: Barnes C, Oliver M, Barton L (eds) Disability studies today. Polity Press, Cambridge, p. 58–76

Hugman R 1991 Power in caring professions. Macmillan, Basingstoke

Humphries S, Gordon PG 1992 Out of sight: the experience of disability, 1900–1950. Northcote House, Plymouth

Hunt P (ed.) 1966 Stigma: the experience of disability. Geoffrey Chapman, London

Hurt JS 1988 Outside the mainstream: a history of special education. BT Batsford, London

Illich I 1975 Medical nemesis: the expropriation of health. Marion Boyars, London

Illich I, Zola IK, McKnight J et al 1977 Disabling professions. Marian Boyars, London

Imrie R 1998 Oppression, disability and access in the built environment. In: Shakespeare T (ed.) The disability reader: social science perspectives. Cassell, London, p. 129–146

Jay P, Mendez A, Monteath HG 1992 The Diamond Jubilee of the Professional Association 1932–1992: an historical review. British Journal of Occupational Therapy 55(7):252–256

Jones K 2000 The making of social policy in Britain. Athlone Press, London

Jupp V (ed.) 2006 The Sage dictionary of social research methods. Sage, London

Kagan A, Duchan JF 2004 Consumers' views of what makes therapy worthwhile. In: Duchan JF, Byng S (eds) Challenging aphasia therapies: broadening the discourse and extending the boundaries. Psychology Press, Hove, p. 158–172

Katz J 1998 Terminal care or terminal carelessness. In: Brechin A, Walmsley J, Katz J et al (eds) Care matters: concepts, practice and research in health and social care. Sage, London, p. 42–53

Keith L 2001 Take up thy bed and walk: death, disability and cure in classic fiction for girls. The Women's Press, London

Kemshall H, Littlechild R (eds) 2000 User involvement and participation in social care: research informing practice. Jessica Kingsley, London

Kendell RE 1975 The role of diagnosis in psychiatry. Blackwell, Oxford

Kent D 2000 Somewhere a mocking bird. In: Parens E, Asch A (eds) Prenatal testing and disability rights. Georgetown University Press, Washington DC, p. 57–63

Kerr N 1977 Staff expectations for the disabled person. In: Stubbins J (ed.) Social and psychological aspects of disability. Baltimore University Park Press, Baltimore, p. 123–130

Kerr A, Shakespeare T 2002 Genetic politics: from eugenics to genome. New Clarion Press, Cheltenham

Kielhofner G 2004 Contemporary foundations of occupational therapy, 3rd edn. FA Davis, Philadelphia

Kim HS 1999 Critical reflective inquiry for knowledge development in nursing practice. Journal of Advanced Nursing 29(5):1205–1212

Knight B, Sked A, Garrill J 2002 Breaking the silence: identification of the communication and support needs of adults with speech disabilities in Newcastle. CENTRIS, Newcastle

Kondo DK 1990 Crafting selves: power, gender and discourses of identity in a Japanese workplace. University of Chicago Press, Chicago

Kusukawa S 2004 Medicine in Western Europe in 1500. In: Elmer P (ed.) The healing arts: health disease and society in Europe, 1500–1800. Manchester University Press, Manchester, p. 1–26

Kvalsing A 2003 Ask the elephant. The Lancet 362(9401):2079–2080

Labonte R 2004 Foreword. In: Laverack G (ed.) Health promotion practice: power and empowerment. Sage, London, p. x–xi

Langan M 1998 The restructuring of health care. In: Hughes G, Lewis G (eds) Unsettling welfare: the reconstruction of social policy. Routledge, London, p. 81–116

Lapper A 2005 My life in my hands. Simon and Schuster, London

Leece J, Bornat J 2006 Developments in direct payments. Policy Press, Bristol

Lee-Treweek G 2005 Changing perspectives. In: Heller T, Lee-Treweek G, Katz J et al (eds) Perspectives on complementary and alternative medicine. Routledge, London, p. 3–32

Levinson F, Parritt S 2005 Against stereotypes: experiences of disabled psychologists. In: Goodley D, Lawthom R (eds) Disability and psychology. Palgrave, Basingstoke, p. 111–122

Lewis G 1998 Coming apart at the seams: the crisis of the welfare state. In: Hughes G, Lewis G (eds) Unsettling welfare: the reconstruction of social policy. Routledge, London, p. 39–79

Lillyman S 2000 Critical incidents as caring moments. In: Ghaye T, Lillyman S (eds) Caring moments: the discourse of reflective practice. Mark Allen, Salisbury, p. 11–18

Lillywhite A 2003 Occupational therapists' perceptions of the role of community learning teams. British Journal of Learning Disabilities 31:130–135

Lovell T, Cordeaux C 1999 Social policy for health and social care. Hodder and Stoughton, London

Lucas V 2003 Why I want you to look me in the face. BBC News Magazine, August 6, p. 4–5

Lymbery M 2006 United we stand? Partnership working in health and social care and the role of social work in services for older people. British Journal of Social Work 36:1119–1134

Lyon J 2004 Evolving treatment methods for coping with aphasia approaches that make a difference in everyday life. In: Duchan JF, Byng S (eds) Challenging aphasia therapies: broadening the discourse and extending the boundaries. Psychology Press, Hove, p. 54–82

Macdonald EM 1976 Occupational therapy in rehabilitation: its history and place in health and social services today. In: Macdonald EM (ed.) Occupational therapy in rehabilitation, 4th edn. Baillière Tindall, London, p. 1–15

McKeown T 1979 The role of medicine: dream mirage or nemesis? Blackwell, Oxford

Mackintosh M, Mooney G 2000 Identity, inequality and social class. In: Woodward K (ed.) Questioning identity: gender, class, nation. Routledge, London, p. 79–114

McKnight J 1995 The careless society: community and its counterfeits. Basic Books, New York

Martlew B 1996 What do you let the patient tell you? Physiotherapy 82:558–565

Maslow AH 1954 Motivation and personality. Harper, New York

Mason M 2000 Incurably human. Working Press, London

Mello-Baron S, Moore A, Moore I 2003 Mental health: new world, new order, new partnerships? In: Horwarth J, Shardlow SM (eds) Making links across specialisms: understanding modern social work practice. Russell House, Lyme Regis, p. 118–131

Middleton L 1999 Disabled children: challenging social exclusion. Blackwell, Oxford

Moore M, Beazley S, Maelzer J 1998 Researching disability issues. Open University Press, Buckingham

Morris J 1989 Able lives: women's experience of paralysis. The Women's Press, London

Morris J 1991 Pride against prejudice. The Women's Press, London

Morris J 1993a Independent lives? Community care and disabled people. Macmillan, Basingstoke

Morris J 1993b Prejudice. In: Swain J, Finkelstein V, French S et al (eds) Disabling barriers – enabling environments. Sage, London, p. 101–106

Morris J, Howard D, Kennedy S 2004 The value of therapy: what counts? In: Duchan JF, Byng S (eds) Challenging aphasia therapies: broadening the discourse and extending the boundaries. Psychology Press, Hove, p. 134–157

Moynihan R, Smith R 2005 Too much medicine? Almost certainly. In: Lee-Treweek G, Heller T, Spurr S et al (eds) Perspectives on complementary and alternative medicine: a reader. Routledge, London, p. 33–36

Mullender A, Ward D 1991 Self-directed groupwork: users take action for empowerment. Whiting and Birch, London

National Centre for Independent Living 2006 The direct payments development fund. Department of Health, London

Nettleton S 1998 Health policy. In: Ellison N, Pierson C (eds) Developments in British social policy. Macmillan, Basingstoke, p. 130–145

NHS Executive 1995 Priorities and planning guidance for the NHS: 1996/97. Department of Health, London

O'Hara J, Sperlinger A (eds) 1997 Adults with learning disabilities: a practical approach for health professionals. John Wiley, Chichester

Oliver M 1983 Social work for disabled people. Macmillan, Basingstoke

Oliver M 1990 The politics of disablement. Macmillan, Basingstoke

Oliver M 1992 Changing the social relations of research production. Disability, Handicap and Society 7:101–115

Oliver M 1993 Disability and dependency: a creation of industrial societies. In: Swain J, Finkelstein V, French S, Oliver M (eds) Disabling barriers – enabling environments. Sage, London

Oliver M 1996 Understanding disability: from theory to practice. Macmillan, Basingstoke

Oliver M 1997 Emancipatory research: realistic goal or impossible dream? In: Barnes C, Mercer G (eds) Doing disability research. The Disability Press, Leeds, p. 15–31

Oliver M 2004 If I had a hammer: the social model in action. In Swain J, French S, Barnes C et al (eds) Disabling barriers – enabling environments, 2nd edn. Sage, London, p. 7–12

Oliver M, Barnes C 1998 Disabled people and social policy: from exclusion to inclusion. Longman, London

Oliver M, Zarb G 1992 Greenwich personal assistance schemes: an evaluation. Greenwich Association of Disabled People, London

Oliver M, Zarb G 1997 The politics of disability: a new approach. In: Barton L, Oliver M (eds) Disability studies: past, present and future. The Disability Press, Leeds, p. 195–216

Oliver M, Zarb G, Silver J et al 1988 Walking into darkness: the experience of spinal cord injury. Macmillan, Basingstoke

O'Sullivan T 2000 Decision making in social work. In: Davies M (ed.) The Blackwell encyclopaedia of social work. Blackwell Publishers, Oxford, p. 85–87

Oswin M 1971 The empty hours: a study of the weekend life of handicapped children in institutions. Penguin, Harmondsworth

Oswin M 2000 Revisiting the empty hours. In: Brigham L, Atkinson D, Jackson M et al 2000 Crossing boundaries: change and continuity in the history of learning disability. British Institute of Learning Disability, Kidderminster, p. 135–146

Øvretveit J 1997 How patient power and client participation affect relations between professions. In: Øvretveit J, Mathias P, Thompson T (eds) Interprofessional working for health and social care. Palgrave, Basingstoke, p. 79–102

Oxlade L, French S 2005 Building an A1 nation. Frontline, December 5:24–27

Palmer N, Peacock C, Turner F et al 1999 Telling people what you think. In: Swain J, French S (eds) Therapy and learning difficulties: advocacy, participation and partnership. Butterworth-Heinemann, Oxford, p. 33–46

Parens E, Asch A (eds) 2000 Prenatal testing and disability rights. Georgetown University Press, Washington

Parr S, Byng S, Gilpin S et al 1997 Talking about aphasia. Open University Press, Buckingham

Paterson CF 2002 A short history of occupational therapy in psychiatry. In: Creek J (ed.) Occupational therapy and mental health, 3rd edn. Churchill Livingstone, Edinburgh, p. 3–14

Penn C 2004 Content, culture and conversation. In: Duchan JF, Byng S (eds) Challenging aphasia therapies: broadening the discourse and extending the boundaries. Psychology Press, Hove, p. 83–100

Pilgrim D, Rogers A 1999 A sociology of mental health and illness, 2nd edn. Open University Press, Buckingham

Pincus T 2004 The psychology of pain. In: French S, Sim J (eds) Physiotherapy: a psychosocial approach, 3rd edn. Butterworth-Heinemann, Oxford, p. 95–116

Porter R 1997 The greatest benefit to mankind: a medical history from antiquity to the present. Fontana Press, London

Porter S 2005 Dictionary of physiotherapy. Elsevier, Oxford

Potts M, Fido R 1991 A fit person to be removed: personal accounts of life in a mental deficiency institution. Northcote House, Plymouth

Pound C 2004 Dare to be different: the person and the practice. In: Duchan J F and Byng S (eds) Challenging aphasia therapies: broadening the discourse and extending the boundaries. The Psychology Press, Hove, p. 32–53

Pound C, Hewitt A 2004 Communication barriers: building access and identity. In: Swain J, French S, Barnes C et al (eds) Disabling barriers – enabling environments, 2nd edn. Sage, London, p. 161–168

Powell M, Glendinning C 2002 Introduction. In: Glendinning C, Powell M, Rummery K (eds) Partnerships, New Labour and the governance of welfare. The Policy Press, Bristol

Priestley M 1999 Disability politics and community care. Jessica Kingsley, London

Prime Minister's Strategy Unit 2005 Improving the life chances of disabled people. Strategy Unit, London

Reason P, Heron J 1986 Research with people: the paradigm of co-operative experiential enquiry. Person-Centred Review 1:456–476

Resnick JS 2000 Work-therapy and the disabled British soldier in the First World War: the case of Shepherd's Bush Military Hospital, London. In: Gerber DA (ed) Disabled veterans in history. University of Michigan Press, Ann Arbor, p. 185–203

Reynolds F 2004a The subjective experience of illness. In: French S, Sim J (eds) Physiotherapy: a psychosocial approach, 3rd edn. Butterworth-Heinemann, Oxford, p. 159–172

Reynolds F 2004b The professional context. In: Swain J, Clark J, Parry K et al (eds) Enabling relationships in health and social care: a guide for therapists. Butterworth-Heinemann, Oxford, p. 17–28

Reynolds F 2004c Two-way communication. In Swain J, Clark J, Parry K et al (eds) Enabling relationships in health and social care: a guide for therapists. Butterworth-Heinemann, Oxford, p. 109–130

Reynolds F 2004d Enabling relationships in group contexts. In: Swain J, Clark J, Parry K et al (eds) Enabling relationships in health and social care: a guide for therapists. Butterworth-Heinemann, Oxford, p. 131–150

Rhodes M 2004 Women in medicine: doctors and nurses, 1850–1920. In: Brunton D (ed.) Medicine transformed: health, disease and society in Europe, 1800–1930. Manchester University Press, Manchester, p. 151–179

Richman J 1987 Medicine and health. Longman, London

Rioux MH, Bach M 1994 Disability is not measles: new research paradigms in disability. Roeber Institute, North York, Ontario

Robson P, Begum N, Locke M 2003 Developing user involvement. Policy Press, Bristol

Rolfe G, Freshwater D, Jasper M 2001 Critical reflection for nursing and the helping professions. Palgrave, Houndmills

Roulstone A, Barnes C 2005 Working futures: disabled people, policy and social inclusion. The Policy Press, Bristol

Roy A, Spinks RM 2005 Real lives: personal and photographic perspectives on albinism. Albinism Fellowship, Burnley

Ryan W 1971 Blaming the victim. Orbach and Chambers, London

Ryan J, Thomas F 1990 The politics of mental handicap, revised edn. Free Association Books, London

Sagan A 1987 The health of nations. Basic Books, New York

Saks M 2005 Political and historical perspectives. In: Heller T, Lee-Treweek G, Katz J et al (eds) Perspectives on complementary and alternative medicine. Routledge, London, p. 59–82

Sapey B, Hughes J 2005 Professional barriers and facilitators: policy issues for an enabling salitariat. In: Roulstone A, Barnes C (eds) Working futures: disabled people, policy and social inclusion. The Policy Press, Bristol, p. 287–300

Schein EH 1985 Organisational culture and leadership. Jossey-Bass, San Francisco

Schlich T 2005 The emergence of modern surgery. In: Brunton D (ed.) Medicine transformed: health disease and society in Europe, 1800–1930. Manchester University Press, Manchester, p. 61–91

Schön D 1983 The reflective practitioner: how professionals think in action. Basic Books, New York

Schön D 1987 Educating the reflective practitioner: towards a new design for teaching and learning in the professions. Jossey-Bass, San Francisco

Schwartz KB 2003 History of occupational therapy. In: Crepeau EB, Cohn ES, Schell BAB (eds) Willard and Spackman's occupational therapy, 10th edn. Lippincott, Williams and Wilkins, Philadelphia, p. 18–31

Scriven A 2005 Promoting health: perspectives, policies, principles, practice. In: Scriven A (ed.) Health promoting practice: the contributions of nurses and allied health professionals. Palgrave, Houndmills, p. 1–16

Scull AT 1979 Museums of madness. Penguin, Harmondsworth

Seligman M 1975 Helplessness: on depression, development and death. WH Freeman, San Francisco

Shakespeare T, Gillespie-Sells K, Davies D 1996 The sexual politics of disability. Cassell, London

Shaughnessy P, Cruse S 2001 Health promotion with people who have a learning disability. In: Thompson J, Pickering S (eds) 2001 Meeting the health needs of people who have a learning disability. Baillière Tindall, London, p. 126–159

Shearer A 1974 Housing to fit the handicapped. In: Boswell DM, Wingrove JM (eds) The handicapped person in the community: reader and sourcebook. Tavistock, London, p. 61–67

Sim J, Smith MV 2004 The sociology of pain. In: French S, Sim J (eds) Physiotherapy: a psychosocial approach, 3rd edn. Butterworth-Heinemann, Oxford, p. 117–140

Simkiss P 2004 Work matters: achieving success in employment. New Beacon, June 88(1031):26–31

Sinclair K 2005 Foreword. In: Kronenberg F, Algado S S, Pollard N 2005 (eds) Occupational therapy without borders. Elsevier, Oxford, p. xi–xii

Sivanesan N 2003 The journey of a visually impaired student becoming an occupational therapist. British Journal of Occupational Therapy 66(12):568–570

Smaje C 1996 The ethnic patterning of health: new directions for theory and research. Sociology of Health and Illness 182:139–171

Snyder SL, Mitchell DT 2006 Eugenics. In: Albrecht G (ed.) Encyclopedia of disability, Vol 2. Sage, Thousand Oaks, p. 624–625

Southampton Centre for Independent Living 2005 Annual report 2004–2005. Southampton Centre for Independent Living, Southampton

Southampton Centre for Independent Living 2006 A brief introduction. Southampton Centre for Independent Living, Southampton

Standing S 1999 The practice of working in partnership. In: Swain J, French S (eds) Therapy and learning difficulties: advocacy, participation and partnership. Butterworth-Heinemann, Oxford, p. 256–260

Stannett P 2005 Disabled and graduated: barriers and dilemmas for the disabled psychology graduate. In: Goodley D, Lawthom R (eds) Disability and psychology. Palgrave, Basingstoke, p. 71–83

Stewart M, Brown JB, Weston WW et al 2003 Patient-centred medicine: transforming the clinical method. Radcliffe Medical Press, Abingdon

Stone E 1999 Disability and development in the majority world. In: Stone E (ed.) Disability and development: learning from action and research on disability in the majority world. The Disability Press, Leeds

Sumsion T 2005 Promoting health through client centred occupational therapy practice. In: Scriven A (ed.) Health promoting practice: the contribution of nurses and allied health professionals. Palgrave, Houndmills, p. 99–112

Sutherland AT 1981 Disabled we stand. Souvenir Press, London

Swain J 1989 Learned helplessness theory and people with learning difficulties: the psychological price of powerlessness. In: Brechin A, Walmsley J (eds) Making connections: reflecting on the lives and experiences of people with learning difficulties. Hodder and Stoughton, London, p. 109–118

Swain J, French S (eds) 1999 Therapy and learning difficulties: advocacy, participation and partnership. Butterworth-Heinemann, Oxford, p. 261–267

Swain J, French S 2004 Researching together: a participatory approach In: French S, Sim J (eds) Physiotherapy: a psychosocial approach, 3rd edn. Elsevier, Oxford, p. 317–331

Swain J, Gillman M, French S 1998 Confronting disabling barriers: towards making organisations accessible. Venture Press, Birmingham

Swain J, French S, Cameron C 2003 Controversial issues in a disabling society. Open University Press, Buckingham

Swain J, Clark J, Parry K et al 2004a Enabling relationships in health and social care: a guide for therapists. Butterworth-Heinemann, Oxford

Swain J, French S, Barnes C et al (eds) 2004b Disabling barriers – enabling environments, 2nd edn. Sage, London

Swain J, Gillman M, Gallagher A et al 2005 Equal access: a new deal? To investigate low take up of health and social services by visually impaired people living in the west end of Newcastle. Unpublished

Talley J 2004 Change, diversity and influence on patterns of health and ill health. In: French S, Sim J (eds) Physiotherapy: a psychosocial approach, 3rd edn. Butterworth-Heinemann, Oxford, p. 7–24

Templeton S-K 2006 Doctors: let us kill disabled babies. The Sunday Times, November 5, p. 1

The Open University 2002 Disability and difference. Programme 1. Audio CD 2. K202. Care, welfare and community. The Open University, Milton Keynes

Thomas C 2002 Disability theory: key ideas, issues and thinkers. In: Barnes C, Oliver M, Barton L (eds)Disability studies today. Polity Press, Cambridge

Thompson N 1998 Promoting equality. Macmillan Press, London

Thompson N 2001 Anti-discriminatory practice, 3rd edn. Palgrave, Houndmills

Timmins N 2001 The five giants: a biography of the welfare state. Harper Collins, London

Tovey P (ed) 2000 Contemporary primary care: the challenges of change. Open University Press, Buckingham

Townsend P 1962 The last refuge. Routledge and Kegan Paul, London

Turner A 2002 History and philosophy of occupational therapy In: Turner A, Foster M, Johnson S (eds) Occupational therapy and physical dysfunction: principles, skills and practice, 5th edn. Churchill Livingstone, Edinburgh, p. 2–24

Twigg J 1998 Social care. In: Baldock J, Manning N, Miller S et al (eds) Social policy. Oxford University Press, Oxford, p. 344–376

Tyneside Disability Arts 1998 Transgressions. Tyneside Disability Arts, Wallsend

United Nations 1993 Standard rules on the equalization of opportunities for people with disabilities. General Assembly Resolution 48/96, December 20

Vasey S 1992 Disability culture: it's a way of life. In: Rieser R, Mason M (eds) Disability equality in the classroom: a human rights issue. Disability Equality in Education, London, p. 74–75

Vasey S 2004 Disability culture: the story so far. In: Swain J, French S, Barnes C et al (eds) Disabling barriers – enabling environments, 2nd edn. Sage, London, p. 106–110

Vernon A, Swain J 2002 Theorising divisions and hierarchies: towards a commonality of diversity. In: Barnes C, Oliver M, Barton L (eds) Disability studies today. Polity Press, Cambridge, p. 77–97

Vernon A, Hughes-Dennis C, Swain J 2001 Evaluating disability equality training: the national picture. University of Northumbria, Newcastle. Unpublished

Vickers A, Heller T, Stone J 2005 Investigating patterns of provision and use of CAM. In: Heller T, Lee-Treweek G, Katz J et al (eds) Perspectives on complementary and alternative medicine. Routledge, London, p. 325–352

Walmsley J 2006a Organisation, structure and community care, 1971–2001. In: Welshman J, Walmsley J (eds) Community care in perspective: care, control and citizenship. Palgrave, Houndmills

Walmsley J 2006b Ideology, ideas and care in the community, 1971–2001. In: Welshman J, Walmsley J (eds) Community care in perspective: care, control and citizenship. Palgrave, Houndmills, p. 38–55

Walmsley J, Johnson K 2003 Inclusive research with people with learning disabilities. Jessica Kingsley, London

Warren L 1999 Conclusion: empowerment: the path to partnership? In: Barnes M, Warren L (eds) Paths to empowerment. The Policy Press, Bristol, p. 119–143

Waterfield J 2004 Professionals and professional work. In: French S, Sim J (eds) Physiotherapy: a psychosocial approach. Butterworth-Heinemann, Oxford, p. 191–204

Watson N 2002 Well I know it is going to sound very strange to you but I don't see myself as a disabled person: identity and disability. Disability and Society 175:509–527

Welshman J 2006 Ideology, ideas and care in the community, 1848–1871. In: Walmsley J, Welshman J (eds) Community care in perspective: care, control and citizenship. Palgrave, Houndmills, p. 17–37

Westcott H, Cross M 1996 This far and no further: towards ending the abuse of disabled children. Venture Press, Birmingham

Whalley Hammell K 2006 Perspectives on disability and rehabilitation: contesting assumptions, challenging practice. Elsevier, Oxford

Willcocks D, Peace S, Kellareh L 1998 The physical world. In: Allott M, Robb M (eds) Understanding health and social care: an introductory reader. Sage, London, p. 80–90

Williams G 1996 Representing disability: some questions of phenomenology and politics. In: Barnes C, Mercer G (eds) Exploring the divide: illness and disability. The Disability Press, Leeds

Wilson AE 2000 The changing nature of primary health care teams. In: Tovey P (ed.) Contemporary primary care: the challenges of change. Open University Press, Buckingham, p. 26–42

Woodward K 2004 Questions of identify. In: Woodward K (ed.) Questioning identity: gender, class, nation. Routledge, London, p. 5–41

World Health Organization 1980 International classification of impairments, disabilities and handicaps: a manual of classification relating to the consequences of disease. World Health Organization, Geneva

Young IM 1990 Justice and the politics of difference. Princeton University Press, Princeton

Zarb G 1992 On the road to Damascus: first steps towards changing the relations of research production. Disability, Handicap and Society 7:125–138

Zarb G 1995 Modelling the social model of disability. Critical Public Health 6:21–29

Zarb G, Nadash P 1994 Cashing in on independence: comparing the costs and benefits of cash and services. Joseph Rowntree Foundation, York

Zola IK 1972 Medicine as an institution of social control. Sociological Review 20:487–504

Index